Published by LUPUS UK (Registered Charity Numbers 1051610, SC039682)
St James House, Eastern Road, Romford, Essex, RM1 3NH

© LUPUS UK 2009

ISBN 978-0-9563572-0-5

Designed & printed by Bob Watkins Artwork, Design & Print

Previously published as:
LUPUS – A GP Guide to Diagnosis - © LUPUS UK 2000

LUPUS

Diagnosis & Treatment

compiled and edited

by

Yvonne Norton MBE

of

LUPUS UK

please visit our medical website
www.medical.lupusuk.org.uk
for more information

Published by LUPUS UK

LUPUS
(SLE – systemic lupus erythematosus)

"If you don't think about it – you won't diagnose it"

- Lupus – probably the classic multi-system illness
- Ninety percent of lupus patients are female
- No two lupus patients present alike
- Fatigue and joint/muscle pain are common
- Patients may present with few or many symptoms
- Lupus is neither infectious nor contagious
- Major organ damage is possible
- Lupus remains incurable ...
- Early diagnosis can make such a difference ...

"If you don't diagnose it – you can't treat it"

LUPUS – Diagnosis and Treatment

Introduction

It is hoped that this Guide to Diagnosis and Treatment will be used as a Reference by General Practitioners and Associated Health Professionals seeing patients who present with a number of symptoms which are not easily categorised.

My thanks go to all the medical consultants and health professionals who have provided the individual chapters for this guide and to Dr. Nicola Erb who checked through the manuscript and gave excellent advice whilst encouraging me to 'keep fighting lupus'.

Thank you also to the patients who kindly gave permission for the photographs to be included and to the donors who so generously provided the funding to enable the book to be produced.

Yvonne Norton MBE
Vice-Chair & Trustee
LUPUS UK

Please note: throughout this guide 'lupus' refers to Systemic Lupus Erythematosus

The authors of the individual chapters will be pleased to offer any advice or further information which may be required by General Practitioners or Associated Health Professionals.

LUPUS UK particularly thanks the following for their most generous donations which have helped make this publication possible:

The Elizabeth Wiggans Memorial Fund (West Midlands)
Aspreva

Chapters & Contributors

Contents

Foreword

LUPUS is an autoimmune disease, a type of self-allergy, whereby the patient's immune system creates antibodies which, instead of protecting the body from bacteria, viruses and other foreign matter, attack the person's own body tissues. This causes symptoms of extreme fatigue, joint pain, muscle aches, anaemia, general malaise, and can result in the destruction of vital organs. It is a disease with many manifestations, and each person's profile or list of symptoms may be different. Lupus can mimic other diseases, such as multiple sclerosis and rheumatoid arthritis, making it difficult to diagnose.

Physicians are often cautious with their diagnosis as they do not want to label anyone until they are certain of lupus. Moreover, a careful review of the patient's entire medical history is necessary, coupled with analysis of results obtained from tests relating to their immune status to provide accurate diagnosis.

The good news about lupus is that the modern day outlook has changed out of all recognition. Provided the disease is diagnosed in good time, in most patients the symptoms can be brought under control and, in increasing numbers, the medication can, ultimately, be stopped.

The last three decades have seen huge progress in research into the causes and treatment of lupus.

I thank LUPUS UK for producing this guide and hope that it will be of assistance to GPs in diagnosing and treating lupus and will help them and other Associated Health Professionals to offer the medical care and support which patients need.

Prof Graham R V Hughes MD FRCP   Hon Life President
The London Lupus Centre   LUPUS UK
London Bridge Hospital
27-29 Tooley Street
London SE1 2PR

Diagnosis of Lupus

Diagnosis of lupus or any other chronic illness may be established using the 5 Step Programme.
1. Review patient symptoms
2. Detailed physical examination
3. Battery of tests
4. Rule out other diseases
5. Time is sometimes necessary to observe the course of the disease

The First Principle in making a diagnosis of lupus is that the individual has clinical evidence of a multisystem disease and several manifestations such as those listed below may be present:

Skin	Rashes, Mouth Ulcers, Hair Loss
Joints	Pain, redness and swelling
Kidney	Abnormal Urinalysis
Lining Membrane	Pleurisy, Pericarditis, Peritonitis
Blood	Haemolytic Anaemia, Leukopenia
Lungs	Shortness of breath, cough
Nervous System	Convulsions, psychosis

The Second Principle is to examine the status of the immune system and how the cells that comprise the immune system are functioning in individuals having a suspicious clinical history. The most useful test is the ANA (Anti-Nuclear Antibody) test, supported by, and in combination with, the clinical history.

The onset of lupus can be gradual with new and different symptoms appearing over weeks, months or even years. The symptoms are often hard to describe and can come and go suddenly, therefore, it may often be that the patient might begin to feel "it is all in the mind". As a consequence, such patients are frequently categorised as hypochondriacs.

The symptoms of lupus fall into two categories, non-specific and specific.

Non-Specific Symptoms
1. **Fatigue** - the most frequent symptom that affects people with lupus
2. **Weight Loss**
3. **Weight Gain** - may be caused by swelling related to organ involvement
4. **Fever** - indication that lupus is becoming active
5. **Swollen Glands**

Other additional problems commonly experienced by patients may be high blood pressure, headaches, vasculitis, increase in hair loss, miscarriage and Raynaud's Phenomenon.

Specific Symptoms

To help distinguish lupus from other diseases, physicians of the American College of Rheumatology have established a list of 11 criteria which, when combined, point to lupus.

To make a diagnosis of lupus the patient must have had at least **four** of these 11 criteria at any time since the onset of the disease.

1. **Malar rash** - fixed red rash over the cheeks

2. **Discoid rash** - red patches of skin associated with scaling and plugging of the hair follicles

3. **Photosensitivity** - rash after exposure to sunlight

4. **Mucosal ulcers** - small sores that occur in mucosal lining of mouth and nose

5. **Serositis** - inflammation of the serosal surfaces – pleura, pericardium, peritoneum

6. **Arthritis** - very common in lupus

7. **Renal disorder** - usually detected by routine blood and urine analysis

8. **Neurological disorder** - seizures or psychosis

9. **Haematological disorder** - Haemolytic Anaemia, Leukopenia, Lymphopenia, Thrombocytopenia

10. **Immunological disorder** - tests on LE cells, anti-DNA and anti-Sm antibodies

11. **Anti-Nuclear Antibody (ANA test)** - when found in the blood and the patient is not taking drugs, it is known to cause a positive test for lupus, being found in <97% of patients, but is not necessarily conclusive

Helpful Hints

Having seen many thousands of lupus patients pass through his clinics, Prof Graham Hughes offers the following 14 criteria aimed more towards diagnostic help and not to classification (as ACR criteria).

1. Teenage 'growing pains'
Growing pains, at least in the UK, is a label widely used for joint pains in teenagers and seems to cover a spectrum of rheumatology from arthritis variants through to lupus.

2. Teenage migraine
Headache, cluster headache, migraine and a strong history of teenage migraine may be of lupus significance, either at that time or subsequently.

3. Teenage 'glandular fever'
Prolonged teenage glandular fever is a label which crops up time and time again in lupus patients and prolonged periods off school in many lupus patients is a recurrent theme.

4. Severe reaction to insect bites
This is a feature of so many lupus patients. Not only are they susceptible to insect bites but often reactions are severe and prolonged - the skin is a major organ affected by lupus.

5. Recurrent miscarriages
Lupus itself seems not to be a cause of recurrent miscarriage but where the antiphospholipid syndrome (APS) is present, recurrent spontaneous fetal loss can be significant.

6. Pre-menstrual exacerbations
Although difficult to quantify, it is believed that significant pre-menstrual disease flare is sufficiently prominent in lupus to be included in this list. All rheumatic diseases are clinically influenced by the menstrual cycle.

7. Septrin (and sulphonamide) allergy
Adverse reactions to these drugs is quite common in lupus and the clinical onset of the disease may have coincided with the use of Septrin.

8. Agoraphobia
Agoraphobia/claustrophobia are often present at a time when lupus disease is active. A history of these conditions can be protracted, lasting for months or even years. In many cases the history is not volunteered or the episodes are in the interim considered unrelated to lupus.

9. Finger Flexor Tendonitis

Arthralgia and tenosynovitis are common features in lupus and although not specific, the finding of mild to moderate ten-finger flexor synovitis is a useful pointer in the presence of other lupus features. It is subtly, yet significantly, different in pattern from other arthritic diseases.

10. Family history of autoimmune disease

As the genetics and statistics of the various autoimmune diseases become better defined, the strength of a particular family history will become more precise. The family history is important, as lupus is genetically determined.

11. Dry Shirmer's test

A 'bone dry' Shirmer's test (levels of eye moisture) points towards one of the autoimmune diseases and in the patient with vague or nonspecific symptoms is worth its weight in gold.

12. Borderline C4

Genetic complement deficiencies have been known to be associated with lupus for over three decades and in the diagnostically difficult patient, especially where a family history is present, repeated borderline C4 levels can be significant indicators.

13. Normal CRP with raised ESR

An important diagnostic aid. A very low CRP in an otherwise inflammatory situation is strongly supportive of lupus or primary Sjögren's syndrome.

14. Lymphopenia

In the patient with non-specific complaints and unremarkable blood tests, a borderline or low lymph count can be overlooked. It can be common in lupus and is certainly worth inclusion among minor criteria.

The Immune System and Lupus

Introduction

Systemic Lupus Erythematosus (SLE or lupus) is a chronic autoimmune rheumatic disease in which immunological abnormalities combine to cause inflammation in multiple organs and systems. This inflammation occurs as a result of the production of large amounts of autoantibodies (antibodies which attack the body's own tissues) and the deposition of immune complexes (antibodies bound to antigen) into tissues. Hence, the mechanisms by which the immune system fails to distinguish between the body's own tissues (self) and foreign organisms (e.g. bacteria, viruses - non self), leading to the production of a wide-spectrum of pathogenic autoantibodies and tissue pathology, are of particular interest. This chapter will consider what the normal immune system consists of **(part 1)** and then highlight our current understanding of abnormalities in the immune system which may contribute to the development of lupus **(part 2).**

1. The Normal Immune System

The immune system provides a highly organised and versatile defence network essential to the health of an individual. There are three major components of the normal immune system.

1. Cells which co-operate to eliminate invading pathogens and maintain internal order.
2. Substances produced by the immune system.
3. Organs closely linked with immune system (through which the immune cells pass).

The Cells of the Immune System

The immune system consists principally of the white blood cells (leukocytes), these have important roles in host defence and the generation of an immune response. White blood cells may be further divided into two types – myeloid cells (including macrophages and neutrophils) and lymphocytes (B cells, T cells and natural killer cells). Blood cells are produced to maturity in the bone marrow, before being released into the blood circulation. The exception to this is the T cell, which is produced in bone marrow but then migrates to the thymus gland (found in the neck) for maturation.

Neutrophils

Neutrophils constitute as much as two-thirds of all circulating white blood cells. Neutrophils are responsive to the presence of acute tissue inflammation. At such sites, the accumulation of these cells effects the process of phagocytosis (the surrounding and digesting of dead and dying tissues, bacteria, foreign particles etc.) and elimination of inflammatory agents.

Macrophages

These cells perform a variety of functions within the immune system. They are particularly effective in the presentation of antigens (various types of material including micro-organisms, foreign proteins and others) to B and T cells (described below) in order to facilitate antibody production targeted to the antigen. Macrophages, like neutrophils, are also important phagocytes.

B Cells

The defining feature of B cells is their unique ability to synthesise immunoglobulin. "Virgin" B cells are produced which are non-dividing. Once mature, these cells disperse into the circulation but have only a short life span (a few days) and most will undergo programmed cell death (also known as apoptosis). The presence of a foreign antigen initiates a process of activation in which a "virgin" B lymphocyte will undergo cell division and differentiation producing "memory" B cells and plasma cells. Immunoglobulin production in plasma cells leads to large quantities being secreted into the blood circulation with high specificity for the antigen.

T Cells

These cells are principally involved in facilitating or suppressing antibody production by B cells. There are two major types of T cells: helper and cytotoxic/suppressor, which can be distinguished by the presence of either a CD4 or CD8 cell-surface molecule. Helper T cells (CD4+) are involved in promoting antibody production by the B cells. Cytotoxic T cells have the ability to kill unwanted cells (such as viral infected cells). Suppressor T cells act to suppress antibody production in plasma cells and are, therefore, important in limiting the production of autoantibodies. Both cytotoxic and suppressor T cells bear the CD8 cell surface molecule.

Antigen Presenting Cells

The capture, processing and presentation of antigen to helper T cells is carried out by antigen presenting cells (APCs). These include macrophages and dendritic cells (which are shaped like an amoeba or an octopus!), found in the spleen and lymph nodes and B cells. This process is important since helper T cells are not able to recognise antigen independently. Instead, antigen must be associated with other molecules (known as MHC Class II) expressed on the surface of the antigen presenting cell. Antigen presenting cells capture and internalise antigen by a variety of methods including phagocytosis (see above). Once inside the cell, protein antigens are processed (cleaved into smaller peptides) and then associate with MHC Class II molecules. These are then transported to the cell surface where they are accessible for interaction with helper T cells.

Substances Produced by the Immune System

Antibodies

These molecules (also called immunoglobulin) are produced by plasma cells. Each molecule is composed of two distinct regions. The first, known as the Fc region, is similar in structure in all antibody molecules while the second, the Fab (a fragment which is antigen binding), provides structural specificity for a particular antigen. The production of an immune complex (antibody bound to an antigen) facilitates its destruction by immune cells such as phagocytes and cytotoxic T cells. Immune complexes involving self-antigens can lead to the destruction of the body's own tissues and, ultimately, to autoimmune disease.

Complement

The complement system consists of a family of proteins whose function is to facilitate the removal of micro-organisms and unwanted cells to which antibody has bound. These proteins are activated in a sequential order and some will bind to an antibody complexed with its target antigen. Activation of the complement system in turn leads to the activation of phagocytes. These cells contain cell surface molecules (receptors) which bind to complement on the surface of micro-organisms and unwanted cells, facilitating their removal. Abnormalities in the complement system (see later) feature in some lupus patients.

Cytokines

These are chemical messengers secreted by cells of the immune system (macrophages and lymphocytes) which act to coordinate the activities of immune cells during an immune response. Different cytokines have different biological effects on immune cells and are important in the process of immune regulation. Lupus is characterised by the production of high levels of various cytokines during active disease (discussed later), which may contribute to hyper-activation of the immune system.

2. The Immune System in Lupus

It is widely accepted that lupus arises as a result of a complex interaction of several factors: genetic, hormonal and environmental. The interaction of these factors in lupus leads to the production of pathogenic autoantibodies, deposition of immune complexes into tissues and, ultimately, widespread organ/system inflammation. This section considers how certain factors predispose an individual to developing autoimmunity and how abnormalities observed in the lupus immune system may be involved directly in the pathogenesis of lupus.

Genetic Susceptibility

The great importance of an individual's genetic makeup to any aspect of health cannot be over-emphasised and genetic makeup has an influence on the development of lupus. *See chapter - Genetics*

Sex Hormones

In healthy individuals, testosterone tends to suppress the immune system while estrogen has an enhancing effect. The predominance of lupus in females over males implies a role for sex hormones in this disease.

Studies in mice that develop a lupus-like disease have shown that sex hormones affect the disease. Thus, treatment of lupus-prone mice with testosterone can reduce lupus-like symptoms and giving additional estrogen can make the disease worse. In human lupus, unique patterns of estrogen production and metabolism have been reported involving increased estrogen to androgen ratios and the preferential synthesis of the more potent immunomodulatory estrogen types. An increase in levels of the hormone prolactin, which also has immunomodulatory effects, has correlated with active disease in lupus patients. In some female lupus patients, pregnancy exacerbates disease activity which may, conceivably, be due to increases in estrogen and, subsequently, prolactin levels.

The Major Histocompatability Complex

Research into the involvement of genes which regulate the major histocompatibility complex (MHC) in human lupus has identified linked groups of genes (haplotypes) which are associated with disease susceptibility. For example, the haplotype HLA A1,B8,DR3 is present in 35% of caucasians with lupus. Antibodies to DNA, nuclear and cytoplasmic antigens in patients also correlate with MHC. It is, however, important to note that any correlations between MHC haplotype and lupus must be understood in relation to ethnic background.

Complement Deficiency

The presence of large amounts of circulating autoantibodies in lupus, which bind to self antigens, gives rise to the formation of immune complexes. Deposition of immune complexes on tissue surfaces can result in inflammation which, if perpetuated, may lead to tissue destruction. Complement deficiency, and thus deficiency in effective immune complex clearance by phagocytes, is a feature of lupus. Complement deficiency in lupus occurs for two reasons. If the disease is active, the complement factors are deposited in tissues like the kidney and the levels in the blood, therefore, go down. Secondly, hereditary and inborn abnormalities of the complement system (a rare condition in lupus) causing an inability to make certain complement components (such as C1q, C1r, C1s or C4), or a reduction in complement receptors in phagocytes have also been identified.

Cellular Abnormalities

Lupus is characterised by an overall shift towards cells supporting humoral (antibody-producing) responses and an impairment of cellular immunity. Enhanced B cell and T helper cell activity, reduced suppressor T cell activity and defects in cellular clearance of apoptotic material by phagocytes are the major cellular abnormalities observed in lupus.

B Cells

An increased number of antibody-producing B cells is observed in lupus patients compared to healthy controls and correlates directly with disease activity. Hypergammaglobulinaemia is a characteristic feature of lupus and is, in part, a consequence of elevated levels of activated B cells.

T Cells

Impaired T cell activation and activation induced cell death, together with increased apoptosis of natural killer T cells, have been reported in lupus. A reduction in numbers of circulating CD8 suppressor T cells are observed in patients with lupus and may explain the ineffective regulation of autoantibody producing B cells. In contrast an increase in numbers of circulating T cells providing help for antibody production (CD4+ T cells) is also found in patients with lupus.

Cytokines

Cytokines which promote help for antibody production (such as interleukin-6 and interleukin-10) are elevated in lupus, particularly in patients with active disease. Interleukin-2 production, a cytokine involved in regulating suppressor T cell activity (and thus autoantibody production), is notably decreased in lupus patients. More recently, an important role for enhanced interferon production in lupus has been suggested. A pathogenic role for cytokines in lupus is also supported by studies showing protective effects of neutralising antibodies to cytokines in both mouse models of lupus and in cultured blood cells from lupus patients. Of recent and particular interest, is a report of the development of systemic autoimmunity and lupus-like disease in mice lacking a gene (SOCS-1) critical in the regulation of several cytokines (including interferons, interleukin-6/10).

Impaired clearance of apoptotic material - a possible source of autoantigens

A link between complement deficiency and lupus led to the hypothesis that impairment in the clearance of apoptotic cells and immune complexes deposited into tissues may be important defects in lupus. In agreement with this hypothesis, studies have shown that many of the key autoantigens in lupus are present in surface blebs of apoptotic cells which have not been efficiently removed from circulation by phagocytes. This observation provides an immunopathological model in which inefficiently cleared apoptotic cells provide a source of key autoantigens in lupus which, in turn, leads to polyclonal B cell activation, autoantibody production and immune complex deposition. Inefficient clearance of immune complexes may result in inflammation which, if perpetuated, leads to tissue pathology. This model has led to the suggestion that lupus is "a disease of defective waste disposal".

Autoantibodies

A wide spectrum of circulating antibodies which bind to self targets (particularly DNA) are found in patients with lupus. Autoantibodies to a variety of antigens (including nuclear, cytoplasmic and plasma membrane antigens) have been identified and some of these may be involved in tissue damage. Antibodies to double-stranded DNA are a hallmark of active lupus and appear to be involved in tissue destruction. Deposits of these antibodies alone or complexed with nucleosomes (DNA bound to histone proteins) have been identified in kidney biopsies from patients with glomerulonephritis, which has resulted from a previous local immune response leading to inflammation.

Summary

The clinical features of lupus are the consequence of its complex immunopathology, a combination of genetic, hormonal and environmental factors. The interaction of these factors leads to the production of pathogenic autoantibodies and the formation of immune complexes. Inappropriate control of cell mediated immune responses leads to ineffective clearance of autoantibody and immune complexes and possible widespread tissue and organ damage.

Figure I. An overview of the normal immune system response

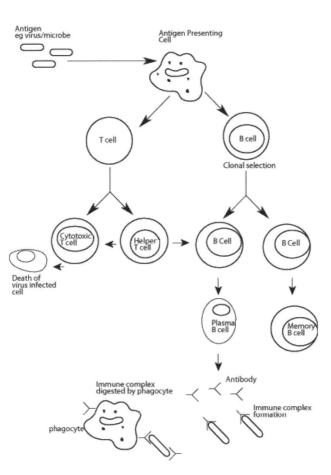

Dr Barry Ripley
Prof David Latchman
Medical Molecular Biology Unit
UCL Institute of Child Health London

Prof David Isenberg
The Centre for Rheumatology
University College London

Genetics

Introduction

There is no doubt that lupus runs in families suggesting a genetic contribution to the disease. Family members of a patient with lupus have an estimated 3-10% chance of developing the disease themselves although, frequently, it is not lupus that develops but another connective tissue disease such as Sjögren's Syndrome or MCTD. Amongst identical twins the risk of lupus rises to 25%. The fact that the penetrance is not 100% suggests strongly that factors other than genetics are important in the development of the disease. Such factors could be either environmental or random. Random genetic events include recombination of T cell receptor and immunoglobulin genes which may contribute to the pathogenesis of the disease. This theory would be concordant with the observation that most twin studies have shown that the time of onset of disease can vary enormously between identical twins even though they effectively have identical genetic makeup and are exposed to the same environmental agents. The genes which are now known to be important in predisposing towards lupus are the DR genes, the complement genes, the X chromosome and race.

DR Genes

The DR genes are a set of polymorphic sequences located on chromosome 6. They are critically important in presenting antigen to responding T cells and there is now increasing evidence that different DR genes have particular preferences for different antigens. A number of epidemiological studies have examined associations between DR and lupus and all are agreed that DR2 and DR3 are increased compared to the general population. The reason for this association is not clear. Work from the late '70s has suggested that patients who are DR3 positive, in particular, have defective clearance of immune complexes, although more recent work suggesting a specific binding of individual peptides of autoantigens may be more important.

Complement

Complement has a central role in the pathogenesis of lupus. Patients with homozygous complement deficiencies have a very high frequency of lupus. For example, lupus or lupus-like syndromes occur in 80% of patients with total C1q deficiency, approximately 60% of those with C2 deficiency and about 30% of patients with C4 deficiency. Although the risk of lupus in patients with complement deficiency is high, C1q deficiency and C2 deficiency is extremely rare, with less than 100 patients with each being described in the world literature. Thus, it is extremely unlikely that the average patient will have a "knockout" for one of these genes. The role for complement deficiency in the pathogenesis in lupus has now been clarified by the "garbage disposal hypothesis".

This hypothesis is based on the observation that complement components are important in the clearance of material from apoptotic or necrotic cells. Cell death results in the exposure of nuclear antigens, including DNA, nucleosomes and ribonuclear proteins, to the immune system. Therefore, the characteristic pattern of autoimmunity in lupus (antinuclear antibodies) is due, at least in part, to the failure to remove nuclear antigens due to the defective removal of cellular "garbage". Other clearance mechanisms including DNAse and C-reactive protein are also defective in patients with lupus and the genetic basis for these has been demonstrated in animal models. Complement is also important in the clearance of immune complexes which themselves are thought to be involved in the pathogenesis of disease. The complement gene, C4, has two different loci, C4a and C4b. Absence of one of the loci, C4a, is quite common in the healthy population and is considerably more common in patients with lupus. However, those who lack this gene on one chromosome almost always have it on the other. In addition, any patients with C4a deficiency are likely to have both copies of C4b, so true C4 deficiency is extremely rare. The C4a null gene, however, is more common in lupus compared to the normal population though this may be because the C4 loci also lie on chromosome 6 and C4a null is in linkage disequilibrium with DR3.

Female sex

Lupus is approximately 9 times more common in women than men, though evidence suggests that this is due to an indirect effect associated with sex hormones rather than the presence of two X chromosomes. Lupus is uncommon before the menarche and, in most cases, also relatively mild when it occurs post-menopausally. Both in vitro and work in animal models suggest that estrogens, in particular, have a pro-inflammatory effect and are liable to make lupus worse, whereas the opposite is observed with androgens and, to a lesser extent, progesterones. Apart from conferring risk, the implication of this is that hormone replacement therapy (HRT) and oral contraceptives should be used with extreme caution with patients with lupus, though some recent studies have suggested that HRT is safe in patients with late onset disease. It is also possible that progesterone-only pills have a weak therapeutic effect providing they are tolerated.

Ethnic groups

Lupus is approximately 4 times more common in Afro-Caribbeans than in Western Caucasians. Precise figures are not available but it is likely that the same holds for Oriental races, particularly those derived from equatorial islands such as the Philippines and the Seychelles. In contrast to this, the frequency of lupus in rural Africa is reported to be low with a higher frequency in urban African populations. This is now thought to be due to interbreeding between different races, which has occurred particularly on tropical island populations, which result in a mixture of different risk factor genes being aggregated into the same population.

Conclusion

Although much remains unknown about genetic factors predisposing to lupus, there is no doubt that it is a polygenic rather than monogenic disease. As a rare disease, its relative risk is increased when there is an affected member of the family. However, it is still not considered worthwhile to screen all family members for evidence of lupus, particularly as some studies have shown that unaffected family members can be antinuclear antibody positive, in which case screening tests are difficult to interpret. Nevertheless, the familial tendency is such that any manifestations which could be interpreted as being due to lupus should be taken seriously and it should be considered as a possible diagnosis if another family member is affected. It is always worthwhile seeking a family history of other autoimmune diseases which may or may not be related to lupus. Sjögren's Syndrome is strongly associated with lupus and organ specific autoimmune diseases, such as thyroid disease and diabetes, are more common in families with lupus, probably because they are also associated with the DR3 gene.

In conclusion, family history of lupus or other autoimmune diseases, including organ-specific disease, should point the clinician towards lupus in the patient with the realisation that it is not, as such, genetic but a disease in which risk factors are inherited.

Prof Patrick Venables
Kennedy Institute of Rheumatology
1 Aspenlea Road
Hammersmith
London W6 8LH

Epidemiology of Lupus

Rates of Occurrence and Risk Factors

Introduction

Lupus (Latin for 'wolf'), was first coined as a medical term in the 18th Century to describe a variety of skin conditions. In the early 21st century, systemic lupus erythematosus (SLE) is recognised as a chronic, often-severe autoimmune rheumatic disease that affects people worldwide. With the evolution of immuno-logical understanding, including the recognition of the antinuclear factor, and the development of American College of Rheumatology criteria for the classification of lupus, more studies have been carried out allowing a deeper understanding of occurrence, epidemiology and risk factors.

Prevalence and Incidence

Lupus appears to be a relatively uncommon disease. The prevalence has been estimated in several different countries mostly, however, in the developed world, using different techniques of case ascertainment. The authors of one meta-analysis (including those studies in Europe and North America) suggested an overall weighted mean prevalence of 24/100,000 population. Three English studies have produced prevalence estimates of: 12/100,000, 25/100,000 and 28/100,000 and the only study in N Ireland estimated a rate of 254/100,000. Studies in countries which include predominantly white populations have resulted in lower prevalence estimates (e.g. England) when compared with studies among populations with a significant proportion of Afro-Caribbeans, Asians and Hispanics.

It is more difficult to estimate incidence for a rare disease but studies in both North America and Europe have produced estimates that are similar (approxi-mately 1 - 8 cases per 100,000 persons per year). The lowest rates of incidence were seen among Caucasian Americans, Canadians and Spaniards and the highest rates among Asian (10.0 cases /100,000) and Afro-Caribbean (21.9 cases /100,000) residents of the UK. In an average UK practice list of 3000 patients, therefore, a GP would not expect to see a new case of lupus more often than every 7-10 years.

Gender

Lupus occurs primarily in women, in particular during childbearing years, when approximately 9 of 10 cases of lupus are female. Female gender is the single strongest host factor in predicting occurrence of lupus. Although still evident in childhood and late-onset lupus, the female predominance rises with puberty, peaking in young adulthood and then declines after the female menopause. The reasons for this gender imbalance are not currently known, but genetic, hormonal and differential exposure to occupational and environmental factors may be relevant.

Age

Although the age-adjusted prevalence and incidence rates obtained in the epidemiological studies are not homogeneous, the peak age of onset among women seems to be during childbearing years, between 15 and 40 years. Importantly however, the median age at diagnosis among women is 37-50 years across these studies, reflecting that this is frequently a delayed diagnosis. Lupus with age at onset > 50 years has been shown to have slightly lower disease activity compared with onset below 50 years of age.

Ethnicity

Whilst lupus is found worldwide, it is more commonly found in some countries, and within a country certain ethnic groups appear to be more susceptible to developing lupus than others. Additionally, the course and presentation of lupus appears to vary between patients of different ethnicities.

In the UK, lupus was more prevalent among people of Afro-Caribbean origin, followed by Asians and then Caucasians. Similarly, studies among populations in Australia and New Zealand found higher rates of occurrence among aboriginals when compared with Caucasians and studies in China, the Philippines and Japan all find higher rates among these populations than Caucasians. Interestingly, where lupus has been investigated in West African countries (the origin of the ancestors of many of the European and North American immigrant populations), rates of occurrence appear to be low. It is noteworthy, however, that in most of these studies the non-Caucasians are ethnic minorities within a country and not distinct ethnic groups. For example, Asians within the UK are different groups of individuals representing much biological, environmental and genetic hetero-geneity. In many parts of the world, particularly North America, minority population groups are often socioeconomically disadvantaged. Socioeconomic factors affect access to healthcare, quality of care and compliance with care and it may be that differences between minority and majority ethnicities may be exaggerated by these factors.

Ethnicity does not seem to purely affect the rate of occurrence of disease but also the clinical presentation and autoantibody profile, such that black patients with lupus seem to be more commonly affected by discoid skin lesions, cellular casts in the urine and serositis. Immunologically, black patients are more likely to have a pattern of Sm and RNP antibodies than white patients and anti-Ro antibodies are seen more frequently in Southern Chinese and North Africans. There is evidence that lupus nephritis is more prevalent in African and Hispanic

Americans as well as Chinese and other Asians. The mortality attributed to lupus in the US shows a less favourable outcome for African-American patients and this has been mirrored in British studies. Rates of survival have markedly increased in the developed world in the past few decades but poorer survival continues to be recorded in India and amongst Black Caribbean patients. Again, it is unclear whether this reflects heterogeneous disease presentation or other factors such as inequity of care and socioeconomic factors.

Genetic factors

Lupus has long been considered to have a genetic predisposition. Cases of lupus cluster within families such that a female first-degree relative of a lupus patient may carry a risk increased by up to 6-fold of developing the disease herself. Surveys among twins have demonstrated a high concordance for the diagnosis of lupus among monozygotic twins (24-69%) compared with <10% concordance among dizygotic twins. Additionally, one study showed a striking concordance for the clinical and immunological manifestations of lupus among monozygotic twins when compared with non-twin sib pairs. The authors did, however, reflect that 'behaviour as well as biology' could explain the short interval in diagnosis between twin pairs – 50% of concordant pairs had sought care because of the recent diagnosis in their twin.

The results of many genetic studies suggest a polygenic mode of inheritance for lupus, with possibly as many as 100 genes involved in susceptibility, but perhaps involving 3-4 dominant alleles. Attention has focussed on the HLA (Human Leukocyte antigen) for detailed analysis of genetic epidemiology. These studies suggest that it is Class II antigens (HLA-DR2 and DR3) which are most important among lupus patients but with different strengths of association in different racial groups. One group has investigated an 'autoimmunity' gene among multi-case families and have proposed an autosomal dominant pattern of inheritance of this gene, with its expression modified by age and gender (higher penetrance in females than males). Polymorphisms in genes for interferon regulatory factor 5 and protein tyrosine phosphatise N22 have been found to be associated with increased risk of lupus.

Hormonal factors

Due to the strong link between gender and lupus, hormonal factors are strongly implicated in the aetiology of the disease. Investigators have explored the role of endogenous and exogenous hormonal factors. Age at menarche may be a marker of estrogen exposure and has been examined as a risk factor in several studies. Although the results are in some cases conflicting, these studies provide some evidence of an increased risk of incident lupus, such that women with a menarche aged < 10 years had an approximate doubling in their relative risk of incident lupus. Menstrual irregularity (long and short cycles) was associated with lupus in two studies but this association was not found in other studies. Age at first intercourse has not been found to be associated. History of miscarriage was associated with lupus but this may reflect the relationship between lupus and the antiphospholipid antibody syndrome. Studies have produced conflicting results in exploring the role of oral contraceptives and lupus. The one study which demonstrated a positive association between the oral contraceptive and lupus involved exposure to relatively higher does of estrogen than those currently utilised and one study suggested a decreased risk of lupus amongst those who used the progesterone-only pill. There is an increased risk of lupus seen among postmenopausal women who had a surgical menopause, with an effect almost entirely explained by use of HRT. The findings of one recent study have suggested that Hormone Replacement Therapy (HRT) can be safely used among patients with known lupus without an increased risk of disease flares.

Socioeconomic factors

Socioeconomic status could have a major impact on lupus disease manifestations and mortality, independent of ethnicity. Access to healthcare, quality of care and compliance with care are all affected by these factors. Few studies have examined socioeconomic status in sufficient detail to truly understand its role in disease development or causation and this is an area requiring further research.

Dietary factors

Nutrition has had little study as an aetiological factor in lupus. Better studied have been the effects of dietary factors among patients with known lupus on disease control. Omega-3 fatty acids are thought to provide a beneficial effect with some anti-inflammatory efficacy. Anti-oxidants (vitamins A, C E and beta-carotene) may also have a positive effect on disease activity. Lower levels of vitamin D have been observed in lupus patients, but it is unclear whether this is because of disease activity. Although nutritional factors may have been poorly studied, this has not prevented considerable coverage in the popular press and on the internet, most of the claims being unsubstantiated

Cigarette smoking

Cigarette smoking has been causally linked to the development of multiple autoimmune diseases, including lupus. There have been a number of hetero-geneous studies of cigarette smoking and lupus which suggest that the risk is modestly increased among current cigarette smokers, as compared with patients who have never smoked. In one study, current smoking was associated with a four-fold increased risk of positive dsDNA antibodies among lupus patients. Smoking may cause DNA damage, promoting the formation of anti-dsDNA antibodies, with a risk that reduces after cessation of smoking.

Alcohol consumption

Conflicting results have been produced with some studies suggesting a protective effect of increased alcohol consumption and others the opposite and yet more suggesting no association at all. These results may well be explained by differences in study design, selection bias, recall bias or uncontrolled confounding.

Virology

Lupus is recognised as being caused by a complex immune autoactivation state, interaction of genetics, selected autoantibodies and other factors. Although concordance is high among monozygotic twins, it is not 100% so, clearly, environmental factor(s) play a significant role in disease development. Despite significant research over several decades, no consistent relationship has been seen between any one virus, or group of viruses, and the occurrence of lupus. Some work with the Epstein Barr Virus (EBV) have shown an immunological structural relationship between Epstein-Barr nuclear antigen-1 and Ro, suggesting that EBV infection might be required before some patients can develop lupus. Serological studies among children and adults support a possible association and experiments have shown that the blood-born viral load is 10 - 100-fold higher in lupus patients when compared with controls. Although consistent with an association, these studies do not specifically implicate EBV in the aetiology or development of lupus. Other studies have explored the role of Cytomegalovirus (CMV), Herpes Zoster and Human Retroviruses (HIV and HTLV-1) and have shown some results to implicate these viral agents in the aetiology but results are currently inconclusive. It may be that infection with one or more viral agents is necessary, but perhaps not sufficient, to cause lupus and that it is the host response or the variation in viral strains that contributes to the risk of the disease.

Immunisations

There are numerous case reports of lupus exacerbation and onset with vaccination against pneumococcus, tetanus, Haemophilus B, hepatitis B and influenza. It is, however, unclear whether this is publication bias or a true association.

Drugs

The phenomenon of drug-induced lupus has been recognised as a lupus-like illness induced by environmental conditions. It has been recognised in association with more than 80 drugs (e.g. minocycline, hydralazine, procainamide, isoniazid, quinidine, chlorpromazine, methyldopa) but behaves differently from SLE. The age of onset is usually older, with men affected equally to women and Caucasians more than other ethnicities. Risk factors have been identified for the development of drug-induced lupus: slow acetylator status, female gender and HLA haplotypes. The prognosis is generally favourable.

Occupational exposures

Epidemiological studies and experimental research have suggested a role for some occupational exposures in lupus. Exposure to silica, solvents, metals and pesticides have all been studied. Silica has been shown to result in increased production of pro-inflammatory cytokines in animal studies and there is a strong body of epidemiological research suggesting increased risk of lupus among those exposed to silica. Work on solvents e.g. aromatic amines, pesticides and metals have not produced clear evidence for or against an association. The relevance of chemicals and drugs to the aetiology of most cases of lupus remains unknown.

Dr Karen Walker-Bone
Senior Lecturer (Honorary Consultant) in Rheumatology
Brighton & Sussex Medical School
University of Sussex
Brighton
East Sussex BN1 9PX

Testing for Lupus

Introduction

Diagnosis of lupus can be made largely on clinical grounds guided by criteria such as those of the American College of Rheumatology (ACR). Routine haematological and biochemical tests in combination with imaging are used to support clinical suspicion of lupus and for monitoring disease activity. In more recent years, in parallel with increased understanding of the pathogenesis of lupus, more diagnostic specialised autoantibody tests have become available. Many of these are used in classifications of lupus and related conditions.

Specifically investigations can be performed to:
- Categorise symptoms into a diagnosis
- Give a guide to prognosis
- Monitor disease activity, either to support clinical findings or to predict relapse.

The precision of a test varies considerably and can be quantified by its sensitivity, specificity, or predictive value. Tests may predict disease activity or relapse and correlate with organ involvement. Ideally, they are also inexpensive, widely available, standardised to other laboratories and allow rapid turnover and results.

Summary of tests:

Routine laboratory tests	Autoantibody & specialist testing
(available to all hospitals and GPs)	• Antinuclear antibodies (ANA) *
• FBC and differential WCC	• Antibodies to double stranded DNA
• U & E (inc creatinine)	(anti-dsDNA)*
• CRP and ESR	• Antiphospholipid antibodies *
• Serum albumin	• ENAs: e.g. Anti Smith (Sm) antibodies †
• Serologic test for syphilis	• Rheumatoid factor (Rh f)*
• Urinalysis (inc 24 hr collection	• Lupus anticoagulants*
or protein:creatinine ratio)	• Anti-Histone antibodies†
	• Complement levels (total hemolytic
	complement [CH50], C3, and C4) †
	• Anti-C1q antibodies †
	† Usually specialist centres only
	* Most large hospital immunology labs

Routine laboratory tests

Routine laboratory tests are an inexpensive way of supporting suspicion of an inflammatory process such as lupus and indicating that further investigation is required. They are also useful in monitoring the level of disease activity and progression in patients already diagnosed with lupus, identifying specific organ involvement (e.g. lupus nephritis) and for the guidance of safe treatment with potentially toxic medications.

Patients on disease modifying drugs (such as mycophenolate mofetil, azathioprine, cyclosporine and tacrolimus) should have regular FBC, U&E and LFT (including amylase) analysis in addition to drug levels in the latter. For example, on alternative weeks after initiation, alteration of treatment or during acute illness, and approximately three-monthly after stabilisation or earlier if any symptoms suggestive of toxicity arise. Regimens for drug monitoring will vary, however, depending on the drug/dose.

ACR Criteria (1997 update)
• Photosensitivity
• Malar rash
• Discoid rash
• Oral ulcers
• Arthritis
• Pleuritis or Pericarditis
• Renal disorder
Proteinuria or cellular casts
• Neurological disorder
• Haematological disorder
Haemolysis, cytopenia
• Immunological disorder
Anti-dsDNA, anti-Sm,
antiphospholipid antibodies
• Antinuclear antibody
(abnormal titre)
[Hochberg 1997]

However, in all such cases and particularly where values are found to be abnormal, the most recent local or national guidelines should be followed, for example those published by the British Society of Rheumatology include guidelines for monitoring second line drugs [BSR 2008]. In some cases, this may mean withholding treatment until discussed with a rheumatologist e.g. in the presence of neutropenia.

Full blood count (FBC)

Lupus patients may demonstrate depletion of all blood cell types and sometimes as part of a pancytopenia. Anaemia is common and typically normochromic and normocytic (the anaemia of chronic disease) but may be microcytic due to iron deficiency (this may be secondary to NSAID/steroid induced GI bleeding). In addition, macrocytosis may be caused by megaloblastic anaemia such as in methotrexate-induced folate deficiency (hence concurrent administration of folic acid is recommended with methotrexate treatment) or from administration of azathioprine. When assessing the relevance of MCV in anaemia the variation from the mean red cell size measured by red cell distribution width (RDW) can give additional guidance. For example, MCV may be normal but RDW increased where there is a combined picture (e.g. haemolysis and iron deficiency) due to populations of both large and small red cells respectively.

Haemolysis (with positive Coombs test*) may give a microcytic anaemia with spherocytosis but, if compensated, may lead to a raised MCV secondary to a reactive reticulocytosis (large immature red cells with prominent ribosomal RNA). If haemolysis is suspected clinically (jaundice, dark urine), a haemolytic screen should be undertaken, including blood film to identify reticulocytes and haptoglobin levels which, in transporting free Haemoglobin to the spleen, will be diminished if red cell lysis is occurring in the circulating blood volume.

Haemolysis in lupus may occur in association with thrombocytopenia. This is most commonly recognised as thrombocytopenic purpura (TTP) or haemolytic uraemic syndrome (HUS) which can be classified under an umbrella diagnosis of Thrombotic Microangiopathic Haemolytic Anaemia (TMHA). Although traditionally thought to be rare, there is now recognition that under-diagnosis is common and its role in lupus gaining increased interest in the literature. It should be considered in patients presenting with these features alongside fever and neurological or renal involvement. This condition is associated with antibodies to CD36 – a glycoprotein expressed on the membranes of platelets and microvascular endothelium leading to debate in the literature about the role for microvascular thrombosis in pathogenesis. A moderate thrombocytopenia (PLT~100) is also seen in APS.

Other blood cell populations affected by lupus include leukocytes, which are typically diminished, lymphopenia being the most common picture. One must also be cautious of a decreased lymphocyte count in Afro-Caribbeans – which might be the result of increased lupus activity or merely the result of an 'ethnic' lymphopenia. This is particularly important given the increased prevalence of lupus in such populations.

Iatrogenic leukopenia is also common, for example, with immunosuppressive drugs such as cyclophosphamide, which may result in acute or chronic myelosuppression. Neutropenia is typical and may be clinically important, but a diminution in total WCC may also reflect lymphopenia, with relative preservation of the neutrophil count. In this situation, it may be inappropriate to reduce or stop a cytotoxic drug, as the lymphopenia may be an indicator of enhanced lupus activity. If in doubt, specialist advice should always be sought.

Some individuals are especially susceptible to extreme adverse reactions to immunosuppressive agents. Nucleotide polymorphisms resulting in deficiency of thiopurine methyltransferase (TPMT), an enzyme responsible for s-methylation of thiopurines (e.g. azathioprine) can lead to accumulation of excessive thioguanine nucleotides (thiopurine metabolites) in haematopoetic tissues. These can be sufficiently toxic to be fatal – such patients can be treated successfully on ten to fifteen times lower doses.

In addition, patients with Glucose-6-Phosphate Dehydrogenase (G6PD) deficiency are at risk of haemolysis when treated with dapsone. These deficiencies should be screened for before commencing azathioprine or dapsone and tests are now readily available in all large centres.

Consequently, WCC is most usefully interpreted in light of total and differential WCC, paying attention to the trend in white cell count and other clinical features such as fever or local symptoms of infection, particularly when patients are on immuno-suppressive medications.

*The direct Coombs test uses Coombs reagent (antihuman antibodies) to agglutinate washed red cells if autoantibodies are bound to their surface. In vivo, macrophages activated by these autoantibodies on the red cell membrane cause membrane damage leading to formation of spherocytes, which are then prone to destruction in the spleen and reticuloendothelial system.

A blood film may also show LE cells but ANA testing has largely replaced this test.

Urea & Electrolytes (U&Es)

Renal complications in lupus patients are common and deranged U&Es can be clinically silent. It is important to screen for abnormalities in U&Es in all patients, but especially those with abnormal urinalysis. Renal function can be defined formally by measurements of a freely filtered molecule such as inulin. However, estimated Glomerular Filtration Rate (eGFR) calculated from creatinine levels (compensating for race, age, gender and body size – see Table) is increasingly preferred due to convenience and is making chronic kidney disease more readily identifiable. More acute changes in renal function are best monitored with creatinine and electrolyte levels.

Lupus nephritis may present as flares with acutely elevated creatinine levels (acute kidney injury). Rapid increase in creatinine levels in a lupus patient known to have chronic kidney disease (e.g. a persistently low eGFR), may also signify progression from background lupus activity to more severe renal damage. Monitoring of blood pressure is also important in such patients since thrombosis of the renal vasculature can lead to occlusion and, consequently, mesangial ischaemia which itself can trigger angiotensin II secretion and subsequent hypertension.

It is also very important to be aware of the large number of therapies in lupus that can cause renal impairment. Treatment with NSAIDs and ACE inhibitors can lead to decreased ability to regulate renal blood flow in response to haemodynamic compromise by impairing afferent vasodilation and efferent renal arteriole constriction respectively. These drugs should be used with caution if renal perfusion could be reduced.

Stages of Chronic Kidney Disease (CKD)		
Stage	GFR	Kidney impairment
I	>90	Normal GFR + Kidney damage
II	60-89	Mild↓GFR + Kidney damage
III	30-59	Mod↓GFR
IV	15-29	Severe↓GFR
V	<15 (inc dialysis)	Renal failure
UK CKD Guidelines http://www.renal.org/CKDguide/full/CKDprintedfullguide.pdf		

In any case, new derangement of renal function should be carefully considered and represents an opportunity to recognise acute and early chronic renal impairment and should be carefully monitored with further investigation where appropriate. Techniques available include laboratory urine biochemical analysis and microscopy for signs of glomerulonephritis or nephrotic syndrome. Any patient who has suffered from renal disease with their lupus should have life-long review of U&Es, BP and urinalysis 3-6monthly (more frequently during an acute episode).

Urinalysis (inc 24 hour urine collection)

Urinary dipsticks commonly test for protein, blood, leukocytes, nitrites and pH. Positive results of any of these tests can signify renal pathology but contaminating causes (e.g. UTI or menstrual blood) should be kept in mind when appropriate. In such situations, a careful history will often suggest a cause. It is important, however, not to dismiss an abnormal dipstick too readily until the possibility of renal pathology can be confidently excluded.

The presence of haematuria is of greater significance if red cell casts can be identified by microscopy, signifying glomerulonephritis which may represent a flare of lupus nephritis.

Proteinuria is defined as protein excretion exceeding 150mg/day and can be used to quantify the degree of renal impairment caused by lupus or its nephrotoxic treatments. For example, an increase in quantified or dipstick urinary protein loss (supported by decreased serum albumin), may indicate development of a more aggressive form of nephritis in a patient with known low grade/stable nephritis (e.g. membranous glomerulonephritis).

Proteinuria can be assessed by a 24 hour collection where the first urine of the day is discarded and all subsequent voidings are collected including the first specimen of the following day. However, Protein:creatinine ratio is now usually preferable in the quantification of proteinuria (10 x urinary Prot:Cr estimates 24hour proteinuria) due to convenience and cost effectiveness, particularly in primary care.
This is preferably obtained from an early morning, clean catch, 'mid stream' urine sample which is more concentrated. Where there is microalbuminuria, albumin:Cr ratio is favoured.

Severity can be graded as following:

Definition	Protein mg/day	Pr/Cr ratio (mg/mmol)	Dipstick protein
Normal	<150	<15	Negative
Microalbuminuria	<150	Alb/Cr: ≥2.5(male) ≥3.5(female)	Negative
'Trace' Protein	150-449	15-44	Trace
Clinical proteinuria	450-1499	45-149	1+
(Macroalbuminuria)	1500-4499	150-449	2+
Nephrotic range proteinuria	≥4500	≥450	3+
*[Adapted from The Renal Association – UK CKD Guidelines 2006 http://www.renal.org/CKDguide/full/CKDprintedfullguide.pdf]			

Liver function tests (LFTs)

LFTs derangements are usually mild and non-specific but are not uncommon in lupus patients, which can be due either to autoimmune liver involvement or treatments employed. Hepatitis with elevation of parenchymal liver enzymes is seen with NSAIDs (especially diclofenac), aspirin and methotrexate and can also be associated with azathioprine or hydroxychloroquine. Corticosteroids can derange LFTs by causing a fatty liver.

Low albumin may reflect proteinuria associated with renal disease or poor nutritional status in patients with severe multisystem disease. In addition, pancreatitis can occur in lupus patients, potentially following steroid treatment and justifies measurement of amylase levels where there is epigastric pain or malabsorption.

Persistently deranged LFTs should prompt consideration for further investigation with abdominal ultrasound and liver biopsy.

C-Reactive Protein (CRP) & Erythrocyte sedimentation rate (ESR)

CRP is an acute phase protein which has been used as an inflammatory marker with a short half life which responds quickly to the development of an inflammatory state – CRP can be substantially raised within six hours of infection.
The CRP level is, however, not typically elevated by active lupus and remains a useful indicator of an inflammatory response to an infection. There are, however, occasions when lupus flares alone can lead to a moderately elevated CRP (e.g. Serositis) even in the absence of infection.

ESR describes the height of red cells that settles in a defined unit of time – usually one hour. Normal upper limits are 15mm in men and 20mm in women and are typically increased in an inflammatory response such as that seen in lupus or to infection. A patient with 'active' lupus will generally have a significantly elevated ESR (often >50), often in the absence of raised CRP as mentioned above. ESR is, however, an indirect measure of all acute phase proteins and can be elevated in many situations, including anaemia and hypergammaglobulinaemia (common in Sjögren's Syndrome). ESR responds less rapidly than CRP and is also slow to change with alterations in the inflammatory response.

Syphilis serology

Lupus can result in a falsely positive VDRL (venereal disease research laboratory) test for Syphilis. This is due to cross reaction of the test antibody and such results must be interpreted in light of the clinical context with an accurate history of sexual partners/activity.
A positive result should be followed up by more accurate tests such as Treponema Pallidum Haemoglutination Assay (TPHA) and the possibility of lupus should be considered.

Specialist investigations

The literature describes over 100 different auto-antibodies in the sera of lupus patients. These may result from the loss of tolerance to self-antigens, including nuclear antigens or cell surface fragments such as phospholipids. Soluble antigens e.g. complement may also be targeted. The identification of these antibodies using the following techniques has assisted with the formalisation of diagnosis of lupus:

- Enzyme linked Immunosorbent assay (ELISA)
- Radioimmunoassay e.g. Farr assay
- Participation assay
- Passive agglutination
- Complement fixation
- Immunofluorescent assays.

Auto-antibodies are polyclonal – they are of varying 'isotypes', with a range of affinities and avidities to their target antigens. The result is that diagnostic tests vary in their ability to identify the slight variations in these antibodies. Given the hypothesis that autoantibodies might be directly responsible for the pathogenesis of lupus, this polyclonality may also influence disease severity through differences in affinity and avidity of autoantibodies to their target antigens (antibodies with greater affinity might be more destructive). Class switching to IgG is thought to be more harmful than IgM and positive IgG antibodies are generally of greater significance than the IgM isotype.

Of these autoantibodies, most are detectable in fewer than 30% of lupus patients and the tests discussed further are the limited number more commonly investigated. ANA is the most sensitive test for lupus whereas anti-dsDNA and anti-Smith antibodies are more specific.

> Sensitivity - % of pts with disease with positive test result
> Specificity - % patients without disease with negative test result.
> PPV (Positive predictive value) - % chance of pt having disease if tests positive
> NPV (Negative predictive value) - % chance of pt not having disease if tests negative
> (*NPV/PPV is influenced by disease prevalence. Sensitivity and specificity are not.)

ANA – Antinuclear Antibodies

Nuclear antigens are those that have roles in cell cycle function, transcription, translation or as structural proteins. Antibodies against any nuclear antigen are known as antinuclear antibodies (ANA). Direct immunofluorescence against these antibodies are reported as a titre, such that high values (> 1:320 – corresponding to a positive signal when more diluted) are more likely to represent true positives than lower titres (1:40).

The high sensitivity of ANA to detect lupus means that it is often used as a first line test of exclusion in patients with compatible clinical features. A patient who tests negative for ANA at 1:160 or less is unlikely to have lupus. Positive results greater than 1:40 warrant further investigation for lupus and, if appropriate, referral to a rheumatologist.

In selected populations, when ANA titres are high, sensitivity of this test for lupus can approach 100% and specificity about 90%. However, false positives are common, for example, in other connective tissue diseases – and particularly in unwell elderly patients. ANA's are also occasionally seen in subacute bacterial endocarditis, pregnancy, HIV, liver disease, malignancy and Type 1 diabetes mellitus.

A positive ANA test result may include specific details of the nuclear staining pattern*:

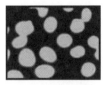 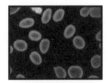 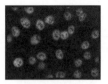 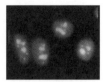

| Homogenous | Peripheral | Speckled | Nucleolar |

- **Homogenous** (nucleosomes) – Lupus, Rheumatoid
- **Peripheral** (anti-dsDNA) – Lupus
- **Speckled** (ENAs) – Lupus, Scleroderma, Sjögren's & Mixed Connective Tissue Disease
- **Diffuse** – Non-specific
- **Nucleolar** – Associated with diffuse Scleroderma
- **Anti-centromere** – CREST syndrome (Calcinosis, Raynaud's, oEsophageal dismotility, Sclerodactyly and Telangiectasis)

(*these are less useful in the context of more recently developed autoantibodies)

ANA is a test with a high sensitivity but with a low positive predictive value since it can be false positive in both normal individuals and those with other connective tissue diseases and so is best applied to those patients with a high predicted risk. Serial measurements are not recommended as there Is poor correlation with disease progression. In addition, lupus-like syndromes are recognised in the absence of positive ANA (other serology such as anti-Ro or La may be positive) and patients with previously sero-positive lupus may not be consistently positive for ANA.

ANA can also be falsely positive in ANCA positive disease such as Wegener's granulomatosis or Churg-Strauss syndrome and these pathologies should be considered if the history is conducive.

Anti-dsDNA – Anti Double Stranded Antibody

One of the most useful types of anti-nuclear antibody to test for in lupus is anti-dsDNA antibodies. These are antibodies found in the cell nucleus, bound preferentially to DNA and are associated with a predisposition to developing lupus. These are commonly detected by: dsDNA ELISA, Farr radio-immunoprecipitation assays and crithidia lucillae immunofluorescence.

Whilst many patients with *active untreated* lupus produce anti-dsDNA antibodies, the sensitivity of this test is limited, with approximately just 60% of patients with lupus having a positive test result. Testing is, therefore, not recommended when ANA is negative, where the probability of lupus would be expected to be low. It is, however, one of the most specific autoantibody tests in lupus – particularly when titres are high and where the antibodies are IgG isotype complement fixing antibodies (rather than IgM antibodies, which precede class switching and are associated with an immature response to antigen).

It has been suggested that anti-dsDNA antibodies might be implicated in the pathogenesis of lupus. It has been shown (using activity indices such as SLEDAI/BILAG), that levels of some anti-dsDNA antibodies appear to correlate with disease activity in lupus and predict flares of lupus nephritis. Furthermore, DNA-antibody complexes have also been isolated from sites of renal damage.

Lupus patients might be expected to be "sero-negative" for anti-dsDNA antibodies early in disease, post-treatment and when the patient is in clinical remission. Anti-dsDNA antibodies are also of less use in subacute or discoid lupus. Isolated negative samples cannot, therefore, be used to exclude lupus. Furthermore, it is recognised that not all anti-dsDNA antibodies are associated with lupus activity - low titres of anti-dsDNA antibodies are sometimes seen in patients with myeloma and, occasionally, those with other autoimmune diseases such as rheumatoid arthritis.

The presence of anti-dsDNA antibodies is generally useful in the diagnosis of lupus, particularly in the context of high clinical suspicion. However, anti-DNA antibodies are heterogenous with different binding characteristics such that some anti-dsDNA antibodies are not associated with clinical symptoms. Anti-dsDNA antibody titres can also be used to guide therapy. In some circumstances, increasing corticosteroid dosage in response to a rise in anti-dsDNA antibodies may pre-empt a clinical flare. However, in most cases, therapeutic decisions should be based on clinical symptoms and signs or other abnormalities, indicating end-organ damage, rather than on changes in anti-dsDNA titre or complement levels alone. Levels of disease activity can often be readily monitored by following a trend in lymphocyte count, climbing ESR or a fall in complement components.

Extractable Nuclear Antigens ENA

These are soluble components of the nucleus and cytoplasm that may be targeted by autoantibodies in connective tissue disorders such as lupus. The presence of a speckled pattern ANA would suggest the need for the following more specialised tests.

Anti-Smith (Anti-Sm) antibodies

Anti-Smith antibodies in high titres are considered pathognomonic for lupus and are included in ACR criteria. They are, however, detectable in as few as 20-30% of lupus patients and are seen in low titres in other diseases. They are most frequently seen in Black Americans and rarely in other ethnic groups. Anti Smith antibodies are targeted against proteins that form part of the common core of U(1,2,4,5) small nuclear ribonucleoproteins (snRNP). Antibodies to anti-Sm(D) are considered most specific to lupus, particularly anti-Sm D1 which are strongly associated with lupus nephritis and correlate with disease activity. Neuropsychiatric involvement is also more frequently recognised.

Anti-Ribosomal RNP antibodies

These antibodies against proteins associated with the common ribosomal core e.g. U1, protein A and C are seen in approximately 30% of patients with lupus and are associated with the presence of Raynaud's phenomenon, whilst also usually indicating milder renal disease.

Anti U1 snRNP

Anti U1 snRNP is most closely linked to MCTD but is also seen in lupus. Its sensitivity, however, is poor and it may be present as part of an overlap syndrome. Testing for anti U1 snRNP should be limited to those with positive ANA, where there is suspicion of lupus/MCTD.

Anti-Ro (anti-SS-A) and Anti-La (anti-SS-B)

Whilst very common in primary Sjögren's syndrome, particularly in the presence of extra-glandular features, anti-Ro and La are also well recognised in lupus where they may be associated with a secondary Sjögren's syndrome with symptoms of Sicca. Antibodies to Ro, a 60 KDa RNA binding protein, occur in up to 50% of lupus patients, especially in the presence of leukopenia, congenital heart block and photosensitive skin rashes.

Antibodies to the 48KDa La antigen occur in 10-15% of lupus patients and predict late onset lupus, but are rarely seen in the absence of anti-Ro. Anti-Ro and La are also recognised in rheumatoid arthritis and polymyositis. Hence, neither is specific for lupus but may be useful in the absence of anti-dsDNA.

Anti-Histone antibodies

50-80% of lupus patients may have antibodies to Histones (which act as intera-calated spools around which DNA wind). This may be to complete Histones or subfractions H1, H2a, H2b, H3 and H4. Specific correlation has been made to drug induced lupus for which there is good sensitivity, but poor specificity – Histone antibodies cannot be used to distinguish between drug induced lupus and systemic lupus, however, drug induced antibodies are usually IgM and may occur without clinical manifestations. Titres usually diminish with resolution of drug induced lupus. This test is probably most useful when interpreting a known history of exposure to relevant drugs e.g. procainamide or isoniazid.

Rheumatoid factor

Rheumatoid factors are usually IgM antibodies directed against the Fc region of human IgG. They occur in 40% of lupus patients but are also positive in a wide range of rheumatological conditions and in the normal population – particularly in older patients. There is also an association with infection, pulmonary disease, PBC, colon cancer or leukaemia. High Titre Rheumatoid factor is a common feature of Type II cryoglobulinaemia (see below).

Lupus anticoagulants and the antiphospholipid syndrome

Lupus patients have an increased risk of thromboembolic disease, largely as a consequence of an association with the antiphospholipid syndrome (APS). Antiphospholipid antibodies are antibodies to negatively charged phospholipids and include the lupus anticoagulant and anticardiolipin antibodies (ACA).

Lupus 'anticoagulants' are antibodies seen in lupus patients directed specifically against plasma proteins (such as ß2-glycoprotein I, prothrombin or annexin V) that are bound to anionic phospholipids. They are so named because in vitro they inhibit the prothrombinase complex, resulting in a prolongation of clotting assays such as the activated partial thromboplastin time (aPTT), the dilute Russell viper venom time (dRVVT), the kaolin plasma clotting time (and, rarely, the prothrombin time)*. In vivo this leads to an increase in thrombotic tendency resulting in, for example, deep venous thrombosis or pulmonary embolus. The presence of APS is also associated with a significant rise in pregnancy related complications.

These antibodies are usually measured by ELISA. Most laboratories report both IgG and IgM titres, but it is elevated IgG ACA that are almost always of greatest clinical significance (compared with IgM antibodies, which are less specific). Diagnosis of the Anti-phospholipid syndrome itself requires clinical evidence of thrombosis in association with the above antibodies. A positive lupus antico-agulant should be re-tested after twelve weeks to confirm antibody persistence.

Cryoglobulins

Cryoglobulins are abnormal proteins that precipitate reversibly at low temperatures and can result in blockage of blood vessels, with subsequent purpura and nephritis. Many autoantibodies seen in lupus behave in this manner. Cryoglobulins may be simply tested by cooling serum in the laboratory. It is necessary that samples be taken directly to the laboratory at 37° (e.g. in a cup of warm water) where the sample can be immediately centrifuged to isolate and refrigerate the serum and hence this test can only be performed in a specialist centre by arrangement with the lab.

Complement

Complement proteins (both free and membrane bound), form an important part of the innate immune defence and are activated by:

a) Classical pathway (immune complexes or CRP)
b) Alternative pathway (bacteria or viruses)
c) Mannose Binding Lectin (MBL) pathway (carbohydrate structures on micro-organisms)

Physiological roles of complement include opsonisation of bacteria, attraction and activation of inflammatory cells, solubilisation of immune complexes and formation of the membrane attack complex with resultant cell lysis.

Deficiency in complement components predisposes to infection, particularly with pyogenic organisms. Deficiency in the classical pathway components specifically, is associated with lupus. This is recognised in the context of inherited complement deficiency and also in the presence of antibodies to specific complement components.

Such findings have led to the hypothesis that complement deficiency is important in the pathophysiology of lupus. This is supported further by the recognition of tissue inflammation and organ damage with activation of certain components of complement (e.g. C1q), in tissue.

Anti-C1q antibodies

C1q is the first component in the classical activation pathway of complement and is thought to be particularly important in the context of severe systemic lupus and lupus nephritis – indeed, antibodies to C1q are closely correlated with damage to the kidneys and more severe lupus activity. C1q may have a role to play in immune complex clearance – it is thought that tissue injury may arise from defective immune complex clearance as a result of hypocomplementaemia.

Defective clearance of apoptotic cells may also underlie such damage. An increasing C1q antibody titre in lupus patients can be used to predict a flare in lupus nephritis – this is of use in both screening and follow up of individuals susceptible to development and progression of lupus nephritis. An association is also recognised between C1q antibodies and hypocomplementaemic urticarial vasculitis syndrome (HUVS).

C3 and C4

All three complement pathways converge at C3, 'the common pathway'. Persistently low C3 levels are seen in lupus patients and may be due to consumption by immune complexes. Binding of the cleavage product (C3b) to micro-organisms and immune complexes results in activation of the terminal complement components, with activation of the membrane attack complex (MAC – C5b-9).

C4 is highly polymorphic and encoded by two genes (C4A and C4B) which differ considerably with regards to their antigenic binding activities. Complete C4 deficiency requires homozygosity for the rare double null haplotype C4AQ0,BQ0 and predisposes to infection and lupus. Partial C4 deficiency is more common and associated with lesser auto-immune phenomena.

Laboratory measurement of acute consumption of C3 and C4 in this scenario can be used to anticipate a lupus flare. Alternatively, a surge in complement degradation products (C3d and C4d) also demonstrate disease activity. It is recognised that homozygous genetic deficiencies in C3 and C4 also predispose to lupus.

CH50

The total haemolytic 50% (CH50) assay represents a functional assay of the activity of the entire complement system, by measuring the ability of a test sample to lyse 50% of a standardised suspension of sheep erythrocytes coated with anti-erythrocyte antibody. This assesses the classical pathway of activation and also terminal components of the complement system. The degree of lysis is proportional to the amount of complement in the test solution.

CH50 is not routinely measured in most laboratories, but it may be useful in the detection of genetically determined complement deficiency (e.g. C1q or C2).

Conclusion

Whilst lupus is a predominantly clinical diagnosis, developments in more specialist tests, particularly auto-antibodies, strengthens the role of investigations in diagnosis. Additionally, the multi-system nature of lupus demands close vigilance of all organs, reinforcing the importance of routine investigations which, alongside serology, are useful in monitoring disease activity. Results should be interpreted in the context of the clinical picture. Better understanding of the methodology and limitations of investigations often facilitates such an approach.

Dr Richard W Lee
Academic Clinical Fellow
    Allergy & Respiratory Medicine
Guy's and St Thomas' Hospitals
London

Prof Kevin A Davies
Professor of Medicine & Honorary
    Consultant Rheumatologist
Brighton & Sussex Medical School
University of Sussex
Brighton
East Sussex BN1 9PX

Research - The Future

Introduction

Research is the systematic investigation into and the study of materials, sources, and the like, in order to establish facts and reach new conclusions. This chapter will address the main areas of lupus research namely causation and new therapies. Although mouse models give clues and insight into disease processes, they are not an adequate substitute for the naturally occurring human disease. Hence, without the generous donation of blood, tissue and time by the patients themselves, little of what follows would be possible.

Factors in the development of Lupus

An extensive search for genetic factors that predispose to lupus have confirmed that lupus is a polygenic disorder and the research challenge is to unravel the complex interplay between gene products that produce the milieu that fosters the varied clinical condition we recognise as lupus.

Lupus is characterised by the production of autoantibodies particularly to nuclear antigens and certain enzymes related to nucleic acid function. Detection of these antibodies in blood is crucial in the investigation of patients suspected of having lupus. The ascertainment that the major auto-antigens involved, namely DNA, histones, Sm, SS-A, SS-B and RNP are clustered in surface blebs on apoptotic cells (cells undergoing programmed cell death) has led to the hypothesis that these surface blebs are critical immunogens in lupus. Furthermore, aberrations in the apoptotic process itself may be central to lupus immunopathogenesis.

It has long been recognised that immune complexes play an important role in the tissue damage, particularly in lupus nephritis, however, there is now evidence of abnormalities in the pathways by which immune complexes are cleared by lupus patients and this has fostered a whole new research front.

The debate concerning which type of lymphocyte is more important in the immunopathogenesis of lupus has reigned for decades and, as all antibodies are products of B lymphocyte derived cells, one might argue that there is no contest. However, this would be premature. The crucial role of the T cell is exemplified by the demonstration of self-reactive B cells in normal human blood - i.e. do they matter? - and the observation that HIV infection may ameliorate lupus presumably via CD4+ T cell depletion. Mouse data also strongly supports the role of the T cell in lupus, as T lymphocyte depletion, by genetic or biological routes, prevents the development of murine lupus. Furthermore, there has been an upsurge of interest in the role of T regulatory cells (CD4+ CD25+) to explain the disruption of immunological self tolerance notable in lupus. These specialised

T regulatory cells appear to be decreased in active lupus compared to inactive lupus and normal controls. This may appear to be compelling evidence for a central role for T regulatory cells, however, the current challenge is to develop reagents to assist in the further dissection of this intriguing observation.

Expansions of certain families of T lymphocytes in the blood of lupus patients have also been identified. Similar profiles of T cells in juvenile onset diabetes mellitus led to the identification of a candidate retrovirus. A viral aetiology for lupus has long been suspected and, despite the technical difficulties, prospects now exist for the detailed and systematic investigation of this subject.

Epidemiological studies in the last decade have identified that the memorable young sick woman with a butterfly rash is less common than the middle aged female with joint pains. Regrettably, in many patients the time from onset of symptoms to diagnosis is several years and earlier diagnosis would be beneficial. Serological tests (antinuclear antibodies and Ro antibodies) can be very helpful in screening for lupus as ANA negative Ro negative lupus is extremely rare. It is also important for patients that their disease activity is accurately assessed so that adequate additional therapy can be introduced when necessary and there is ongoing research into a number of new markers of disease activity.

Management of Lupus

New therapies for lupus are being regularly introduced and old ones refined. The use of certain anti-transplant rejection therapies such as cyclosporine A (neoral) and tacrolimus (prograf) have shown significant benefit in lupus. More recently, another anti-rejection agent, mycophenolate mofetil, has been demonstrated to be a useful therapy, especially for lupus nephritis. Mycophenolate mofetil works by selectively blocking lymphocyte proliferation and, hence, T cell dependent antibody responses. Where in the treatment ladder mycophenolate should be placed will require further careful observation and clinical trials are in progress.

The prognosis in lupus has improved dramatically over the last 20 years and, hopefully, the long term complications of drugs, particularly steroids, will be further reduced by these new therapies. The use of new antagonists of ovulation may protect the woman's ovarian function whilst chemotherapy with cyclophos- phamide is ongoing.

Information given to patients with lupus must be accurate and, regrettably, misinformation abounds. Well designed studies, using appropriate control groups, have now shown that true allergy is not more common in lupus, that stress does contribute to flares of lupus, that smoking is a risk factor and that alcohol may even be protective.

Depletion of B cells in lupus with rituximab (an anti-CD20 monoclonal antibody) is now a reality but its place in the therapeutic arsenal, and the timing of this therapy, needs further clinical research. Biologic therapies to costimulatory molecules, complement (C5b) and cytokines are all currently being considered/tested in lupus patients

Haemopoietic stem cell transplantation and extracorporeal photochemotherapy are two novel treatment modalities that have been used successfully in small numbers of lupus cases. Their application is currently limited by availability of expertise and expense but may offer hope to individuals with disease at the most severe end of the spectrum. The survival after autologous haemopoietic stem cell transplantation for malignancy continues to improve and real possibilities for lupus exist.

The Future

To those individuals who kindly donate to the "tin rattlers" outside the local supermarkets and generously support coffee mornings, research means finding a cure for the disease in question. Sufferers from lupus demand no less, however, the nature of research, especially laboratory research, is that it often poses more questions than it answers. The last 5 years have certainly confirmed this!

Dr Peter C Lanyon
Consultant Rheumatologist
Nottingham University Hospitals

Prof Richard J Powell
Professor of Clinical Immunology & Allergy
Clinical Immunology Unit
Queens Medical Centre
Nottingham University Hospitals
Nottingham
NG7 2UH

The Heart and Lupus

Introduction

At some stage in the disease more than half of lupus patients will develop a heart abnormality. It is, therefore, one of the important clinical manifestations of lupus to detect although, of course, it need not necessarily be serious.

Lupus involvement of the heart may affect all its layers: the pericardium, myocardium and endocardium as well as the coronary arteries. Involvement may be primary or secondary to lupus damage to other organs, such as the lungs. In addition, symptoms may be confused with other clinical conditions such as reflux oesophagitis, pleurisy and costochondritis.

Working step-wise through the layers of the heart this chapter will describe how they may be involved in lupus and what the clinical manifestations are.

Pericarditis

This is the most common heart abnormality in lupus and reports estimate that 6-45% of lupus patients will have some form of pericardial abnormality (it may, however, go undiagnosed).

Inflammation of the pericardium can cause symptoms due to the inflammatory mediators that accumulate and stimulate pain receptors. In some instances a pericardial effusion will occur and sometimes the effects of pericardial inflammation cause the pericardium to constrict, which may cause additional symptoms. An uncommon complication that may occur is for the pericardium to become infected by organisms (usually bacterial) that are carried to it in the blood.

The following symptoms may occur:
• **Sub-sternal pain:** this may be aggravated by breathing, coughing, swallowing, twisting or bending forward. There is a range of severity and the symptoms may be intermittent.
• **Breathlessness:** this is caused because the heart is unable to function efficiently either due to its constriction by the pericardium or by fluid that may collect around the heart muscle.
If a diagnosis is suspected, it can be confirmed by listening to the heart when a friction rub may be heard on auscultation. In addition, characteristic electrocardiographic changes may be present (tall T waves and elevated ST segments). An echocardiogram is useful for visualising pericardial effusions. In the absence of signs and symptoms of a pericardial effusion, fluid drainage is rarely necessary.

Myocarditis

This is not a common problem and estimates suggest that up to only 10% of patients will develop this cardiac abnormality. Acute myocarditis may be associated with a lupus flare, but may be drug induced e.g. due to cyclophosphamide or anti-malarials. Similar inflammation may also be found in skeletal muscles and myocarditis may be part of a generalised myositis. Some reports suggest that anti-RNP antibodies may be more prevalent in these patients. Interestingly, anti-myocardial antibodies have been detected in some patients with lupus but they do not correlate with heart involvement.

Immune complex deposition within the myocardium is also thought to form part of the pathological process by activating the complement cascade.

Clinical symptoms of myocarditis:

- **Tachycardia**
- **Breathlessness**
- **Palpitations**

Signs of congestive heart failure may also be present, with a gallop rhythm and other heart murmurs that may be heard on auscultation. Conduction abnormalities may occur after myocarditis and are usually transient.

Investigations may demonstrate heart enlargement on x-ray and arrhythmias when the ECG is taken.

Endocarditis

In lupus this can be called Libman-Sachs endocarditis. Inflammation of this heart structure results in small nodules (vegetations) being formed. These range from about 1-4mm in diameter and may be singular or conglomerate and have been described as "mulberry-like clusters". They are usually found near the edge of valves but can also occur between the atrial and ventricular chambers. Some reports suggest that antiphospholipid antibodies are associated with valvular heart disease, particularly affecting the mitral valve.

Clinical symptoms of endocarditis:

- **Tachycardia**
- **Fever**
- **General malaise**

Echocardiography can be used to visualise the vegetations and on auscultation murmurs can be heard as the blood becomes turbulent as it passes the vegetations.

Mitral and aortic valves are most commonly involved.

Cardiac auscultation should be carried out at each visit to the doctor and echocardiography is indicated if significant or changing murmurs are detected or if cardiac function is changing. Echocardiography is not required if there are no symptoms or physical findings on examination suggestive of valvular heart disease.

Complications of endocarditis may be heart failure which could be due to the valves working inefficiently as a result of them not being able to close properly or due to valve stenosis, where the valves do not open fully. In addition, vegetations may break off from the valves and cause damage in a number of other locations such as the brain where a stroke may occur, the lungs where pulmonary embolism may result and peripheral vessels which may become blocked. Libman-Sachs endocarditis may be complicated by infection as the endocardium will be predisposed to attack by blood borne organisms. There may also be anaemia as a result of the inflammatory process.

Antibiotic prophylaxis may be recommended for selected patients with lupus undergoing procedures associated with a risk of bacteraemia e.g. dental treatment. Valve replacement surgery or valvoplasty may be necessary if severe mitral or aortic valvular insufficiency develops.

For patients with asymptomatic valve thickening, low dose aspirin may be indicated.

Non-bacterial thrombotic endocarditis involved with systemic emboli should be treated with anticoagulation. Invasive cardiac screening is not indicated in asymptomatic patients.

Coronary Artery Disease

Symptomatic CAD is described in 2-45% of patients with lupus and may lead to acute myocardial infarction. Studies have demonstrated that atherosclerosis may develop earlier in patients with lupus and it has been suggested that there is increased prevalence of traditional risk factors for atherosclerosis. It is thought that autoimmune vascular injury in lupus may predispose to atherosclerosis plaque formation. Rarely is there inflammation of the coronary arteries (vasculitis) which results in occlusion of the vessel.

This means that attention to modifiable risk factors is important e.g. hypertension, hyperlipidaemia, cigarette smoking, obesity, diabetes and sedentary life styles. Some studies have indicated that glucocorticoids may lead to worsening of risk factors e.g. cholesterol, arterial blood pressure and body weight. Whilst hydroxychloroquine has been noted to produce a decrease in plasma cholesterol level. The association with corticosteroid, however, may be associated with disease severity, as patients who receive high doses of glucocorticoids are more likely to have active and severe disease. It is obvious that minimum doses of glucocorticoids, used for the shortest possible time, is recommended. Coronary angiography may help differentiate atherosclerosis from arteritis.

Other abnormalities affecting the heart
ECG Changes

It is estimated that an abnormal ECG is found in between 34-74% of patients. These abnormal tracings may reflect a primary abnormality of the heart itself, such as pericarditis or myocarditis, or isolated conduction defects may occur such as complete heart block and atrial premature contraction. Sometimes, the abnormal tracings may be secondary to other abnormalities in the body, such as an imbalance in the blood electrolytes e.g. a raised potassium level, which could be associated with kidney disease, or the use of drugs such as corticosteroids and diuretics.

Neonatal Lupus Syndrome (NLS)

NLS is a rare complication of lupus pregnancy and congenital complete heart block is one of its features. The presence of maternal IgG anti-Ro (SSA) and anti-La (SSB) antibodies are thought to be associated with damage to the heart's conduction pathways in the fetus. The risk is thought to be between 1-7%. These antibodies should be measured early in pregnancy if they have not already been measured. It has yet to be established if these antibodies are involved in conduction defects that may occur in adult patients.
See chapter - Pregnancy, Contraception and HRT in Lupus

High Blood Pressure

About a quarter of lupus patients will have blood pressure readings over 140/90 at some stage in their clinical course. This may, of course, be unrelated to lupus as it is a common condition but lupus associated causes are kidney disease and corticosteroid treatment.

Treatment of Heart Abnormalities

Sometimes no treatment is required, for example, in small asymptomatic pericardial effusions. If the cause of the heart abnormality is thought to be associated with lupus, treatment should be aimed at reducing inflammation with NSAIDs, anti-malarial agents (e.g. hydroxychloroquine), corticosteroids and sometimes cytotoxic drugs such as azathioprine or cyclophosphamide.

Other drugs may also be necessary to counteract heart arrhythmias (e.g. beta-blockers) or heart failure (e.g. diuretics). If any part of the heart becomes infected then antibiotics, usually given intravenously, will be necessary. High blood pressure can be treated effectively by such drugs as nifedipine and ACE inhibitors. Drugs such as hydralazine, methyldopa and beta-blockers, which may cause lupus-like syndrome, can also be safely used without exacerbating the disease.

It is recommended that all lupus patients should receive antibiotic prophylaxis prior to and during surgery, including dental procedures.

Table I - Chest Pain in Lupus

Chest pain in lupus is a frequent complaint and causes are:

- Heart: Acute lupus pericarditis, coronary artery disease e.g. angina pectoris and other heart abnormalities e.g. mitral valve prolapse
- Lung disease e.g. pleurisy, pneumonia, pulmonary embolism (antiphospholipid syndrome)
- Gastrointestinal disorders e.g. gastritis and peptic ulcer disease
- Musculoskeletal abnormalities: costochondritis or fibromyalgia
- Osteoporosis: corticosteroid therapy may predispose to osteoporosis which could cause rib fractures and vertebral body collapse.

Renal disease: lupus nephritis and nephritic syndromes may be associated with renal vein thrombosis and pleuritic chest pain is a symptom

---

Prof John Axford
Chair of Clinical Rheumatology
Director of The Sir Joseph Hotung Centre for Musculoskeletal Disorders
St George's
University of London and NHS Trust
London SW17 0QT

The Lungs and Lupus

KEY POINTS:
- Lupus causes a number of acute and chronic lung diseases.
- Lupus of the lung is common and can be important in prognosis.
- Symptoms are similar to other serious pathologies e.g. PE or pneumonia.

Introduction

Intrathoracic lupus is common and may involve the pleura, lung parenchyma, vasculature or respiratory muscles, presenting as: Pleuritis and effusions; Pneumonitis (acute and chronic); Bronchiolitis obliterans; Pulmonary vasculitis; Opportunistic infections; Pulmonary haemorrhage, Pulmonary hypertension, Pulmonary embolus (particularly with anti-phospholipid syndrome) and "Shrinking lung syndrome".

It is important to remember that in addition to primary lupus-induced pleuropulmonary pathology, respiratory symptoms may also be secondary to lupus acting on other organs or due to the side effects of systemic steroid or cytotoxic treatment.

This chapter summarises key clinical features and likely treatments of such conditions, commenting where relevant, on how diagnosis can be focused with investigation – whilst this is often radiological, detailed reviews of this nature are to be found elsewhere. Lung findings in lupus have been correlated with clinical symptoms and serological markers for other rheumatological syndromes e.g. Scleroderma or Raynaud's and also Anti-Ssa/anti-Jo-1 antibodies but the lack of evidence supporting their role in diagnosis renders them outside the scope of this chapter. Ultimately, diagnosis and management of lupus lung disease is complex and often requires expert management in a specialist centre.

Pleural disease

Up to 60% of patients with lupus experience pleuritic chest pain at some point. Some are associated with a serous/serosanguinous pleural effusion, typically exudative with a high protein and lactate dehydrogenase (LDH) versus serum (LDH here is, however, lower than in Rheumatoid Arthritis and glucose is higher).

Given that chest signs and symptoms can be relatively common, the decision to investigate will depend on the severity of symptoms and whether they present alongside other features that arouse suspicion of new, significant intrathoracic disease. For example, diagnostic aspiration of a new effusion in the presence of elevated CRP is likely to be useful, more so than in an individual with recurrent lupus related pleurisy which has responded well to anti-inflammatory medications. Pleural biopsy is less useful, being poorly specific and, therefore, rarely performed. It should also be remembered that the presence of lupus does not preclude the presence of thoracic disease of other aetiologies.

Lupus associated pleuritis responds to NSAIDs in mild cases or, where severe, may require increased dose corticosteroids. Anti-malarials are useful for refractory cases. Colchicine may also be useful in acute pleuritis.

Pleural aspirates: Aiding the diagnosis of a pleural effusion†

	Lupus	Rheumatoid Arthritis	Malignancy	Para-pneumonic	Empyema	TB	CCF
Appearance	Yellow	Yellow/ green or debris	Bloody	Turbid/ purulent	Purulent, odourous	Typically small volume	Clear/straw colour
Cytology e.g. PMNs	High PMNs & lymphocytes	PMNs <5000/mm3 RA cells. Typical cytology	Abnormal cells. Mononuclear cells	High PMNs	High PMNs	Lymphocytes, mono-nucleocytes	Rarely PMNs
Protein High if Pleural: serum > 50% (or >29g/L)	High	High	High	High	High	V High >4g/dL	Low (<30g/L)
Glucose (Low if <60mg/dL)	High (>80g/l)	V Low (often <25g/L)	Low	Low	Low	Low	Normal or low
LDH (High if Pleural serum LDH >0.6)	High (<500/L)	High >700 but<1000/L	High	High	High	High	Low
pH (norm 7.6, <7.3 suggests inflammation)	7.3-7.45	<7.2	7.3-7.45 (less =low survival)	7.3-7.45 (Drain if <7.2)	<7.2 suggestive (Drain if <7.2)	7.3-7.45	7.4-7.55
Definitive tests	Pleural ANA High LE Cells**	Rh factor e.g. >1:320	Cytology Tumour markers	Culture	Pus, odour culture	AFB, Tuberculin skin test	Echo, CXR, BNP

*Exudates typically have pleural fluid protein of >30g/L. Where diagnostic uncertainty exists, the presence of one or more of Light's criteria: Pleural fluid/serum protein >0.5: pleural fluid/serum LDH (lactate dehydrogenase) >0.6 or pleural LDH >two thirds upper limit of normal are a sensitive means of identifying an exudate [Light RW 2002]
**Rarely performed clinically   †Respiratory medicine (WB Saunders company limited 3rd ed)

Pulmonary Infection

Pleural disease is often complicated by infection, particularly since lupus patients are generally more susceptible to infection, which can account for considerable morbidity and mortality. A number of hypotheses explain this increased suscep-tibility: defective macrophage antibacterial activity; complement deficiency impairing opsonisation and immune presentation of bacterial antigens; immuno-suppression with corticosteroids and DMARD's; oedema and poor clearance of respiratory secretions providing a fertile environment for bacterial colonisation. Unusual and more aggressive, opportunistic organisms e.g. *Aspergillus, Cryptococcus, Pneumocystis jirovecii (carinii),* CMV and *Nocardia* are, therefore, more likely. Hypocomplementaemic patients also have increased sensitivity to more common organisms such as *Streptococcus pneumoniae* and *Neisseria meningitidis,* both of which may result in fatal infection and should be considered even in low activity.

Tuberculosis (TB) is also more common in lupus and should be excluded if haemoptysis, weight loss or fever persist. TB may also give rise to isolated pleural involvement (see above) and suspicion should be high where systemic upset occurs in 'at-risk populations' and those in contact with individuals with AFB (Acid-Fast Bacilli) positive sputum. A chest radiograph may identify multiple opacities or nodular (potentially cavitating) masses.

In any infection, accurate early diagnosis, with microbiological identification of organisms and sensitivities are crucial, and whilst infection in the presence of other lupus-related lung disease can be difficult to diagnose, this may be aided by a high CRP which, in lupus, is generally not elevated, even in the presence of active inflammation. Prompt "appropriate" treatment is essential to rapid recovery, particularly in septicaemia where "Surviving Sepsis" guidelines should be followed. In hypocomplementaemic patients who suffer recurrent infection there is also an argument for prophylactic antibiotics.

Pulmonary Embolus

Sudden onset pleuritic chest pain with acute respiratory compromise should also arouse suspicion of pulmonary embolus (PE), particularly if the ECG shows sinus tachycardia or right heart strain (classically "$S_1Q_3T_3$"). The incidence of thromboembolic events is increased in rheumatological diseases and particular vigilance is required in the presence of antiphospholipid antibodies (aPL) which strongly predispose to venous thrombosis.

Lupus anticoagulants are so named because *in vitro* clotting is inhibited. *In vivo,* paradoxically, thrombotic events are more common. This occurs due to their activity against plasma proteins such as prothrombin. aPTT is unreliable in these patients, being prolonged in only half of those with lupus anticoagulant and often not at all in the presence of anticardiolipin antibodies (aCL). More reliable tests (such as ELISA for aCL or dRVVT for lupus anticoagulant) should be ordered early in patients with suspected antiphospholipid syndrome or where there are unexplained thrombotic events.

Standard risk factors e.g. smoking, oral contraceptive, malignancy, surgery and immobility may also co-exist in lupus and should be considered when establishing probability of venous thrombosis. Corticosteroids also increase the risk of venous thromboembolism, both acutely and chronically.

Patients in whom there is a high clinical suspicion of PE in the presence of pre-existing lung disease and/or serological risk factors (LAC or high titre aPL), should be anticoagulated pending further investigation (CTPA is usually preferred due to a higher specificity when there is previous/chronic lung damage that renders V:Q scanning less accurate). Long term anti-coagulation is generally recommended in patients with high titre aPL who have had a pulmonary embolus.

Acute Pneumonitis (ALP)

This acute, non-infective, inflammatory lung lesion has been reported in up to 9% of lupus patients and with symptoms such as fever, pleuritic chest pain, dyspnoea and cough is readily confused with other acute lung disease unrelated to lupus, including pulmonary embolus and acute infection. ALP tends to affect the young but may complicate CILD (see below) in older patients. The chest radiograph findings may include lower zone alveolar infiltrates, elevated diaphragm or pleural effusion.

Exclusion of infective aetiologies is crucial and it is often favourable to cover with broad spectrum antibiotics where there is any suspicion of an infective component, pending microbiological culture results (whenever possible cultures of blood, sputum etc. should precede antibiotics). Chills and rigors favour infection and a raised CRP is atypical in lupus and also suggests infection. However, such elevation in CRP may also be absent in viral infections. ALP would also be more likely during a generalised lupus flare such that diagnosis is supported by the presence of nephritis, arthritis, pericarditis and pleuritis. Distinguishing an acute lupus pneumonitis from that of an infective origin can be difficult (see below). Systemic prednisolone is the most common therapy. In-patient assessment in a specialist centre is, however, always indicated.

Acute Alveolar Haemorrhage

Pulmonary haemorrhage complicating lupus is almost identical to acute pneumonitis and may represent the same spectrum of disease. This disease is rare and can range from a mild sub-clinical chronic form to massive life-threatening haemorrhage with a mortality of up to 90%. Patients may have haemoptysis at presentation (one study reported 42%), but sometimes manifestations can be clinically non-specific and include unexplained anaemia, cough and dyspnoea. Risk factors include known lupus, high levels of anti-DNA antibodies and active extra-pulmonary disease. Glomerulonephritis is also often present in these patients.

Important differential diagnoses include anti-GBM disease and ANCA associated vasculitis (e.g. Wegener's Granulomatosis or Churg-Strauss Disease). Pulmonary function test results showing increased diffusing capacity for carbon monoxide is a sensitive test for acute alveolar haemorrhage although it can be technically challenging to perform in severe cases. Increasingly, blood stained samples from bronchoalveolar lavage or progressive chest radiograph in association with a fall in haemoglobin are highly suggestive. Lung biopsies show capillaritis with immunoglobulin or immune complex deposition although, clinically, these are rarely indicated. Treatment options include high dose steroids and cyclophos-phamide and, in severe cases, plasma exchange, although the latter can be hazardous in the presence of thrombocytopenia or coagulation disorders.

Pulmonary function tests in Lupus – do they help?

	Restrictive		Obstructive	
	Intrinsic Interstitial lung disease	**Extra pulmonary e.g. kyphosis, neuromusc**	**COPD** *(Emphysema may show a restrictive pattern)*	**Asthma** *Reversible outflow impairment expected*
TLC	Decreased	Decreased	Normal or Increased	Normal
FVC	Decreased	Decreased	Normal or decreased	Normal
PEFR	Normal (or decreased)	Normal	Usually Decreased	Decreased
FEV1	Decreased or Normal	Decreased or Normal	Decreased	Decreased
FEV1/FVC	Normal	Normal	Decreased	Decreased
TLCO	Decreased	Normal	Normal (may be low in emphysema volume loss)	Normal to High

Subacute interstitial Lung disease

Bronchiolitis obliterans (which may comprise an organising pneumonia - BOOP) presents with more sub-acute symptoms of cough, dyspnoea, fever and constitutional un-wellness. Middle-aged women are most typically affected.

Airflow limitation arises from submucosal oedema with peribronchiolar inflammation and fibrosis, primarily involving respiratory bronchioles in the absence of diffuse parenchymal disease, thought to arise from plugs of fibrous tissue in bronchioles and alveolar ducts. Prognosis is better than that for those with a standard interstitial pneumonia, particularly when BOOP is the diagnosis since there is often an excellent response to corticosteroids.

Whilst chest radiographs in BOOP may show focal alveolar infiltrates with striking air bronchograms, there are often no changes in pure BO where the lung parenchyma is spared. Pulmonary function tests show a restrictive defect.

Clinical and serological markers may also correlate with such chronic lung disease in lupus. Both Scleroderma-like symptoms (e.g. Raynaud's) and Anti-SSa (Ro) antibody seem to be more common with restrictive defects and a reduction in transfer factor. Another important differential is anti-Jo-1 associated myositis/lung disease.

All such patients should be assessed in a specialist centre.

Chronic Interstitial lung disease

Chronic interstitial lung disease (CILD) is well recognised in connective tissue disorders yet, in lupus, is thought to be clinically significant less often than in, for example, RA, Scleroderma or complex myositis associated syndrome. Symptoms include progressive dyspnoea and non-productive cough that may develop insidiously 'de novo' or progress from acute pneumonitis.

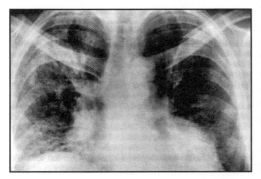

The chest X-ray shows coarse reticulonodular densities in the lower zones but, as with lung function tests, cannot easily differentiate between this chronic picture of fibrosis (due to either cause) and an acute alveolitis – this requires serial investigations. High-resolution CT images can detect such progressive parenchymal change more readily. 'Ground glass', focal alveolar opacities, imply active inflammation, potentially treatable with steroids, whereas macroscopic, honeycomb-like cysts are more consistent with end-stage irreversible fibrosis. CT may, therefore, have a greater Prognostic significance and correlate more closely with abnormal lung function tests, although not necessarily clinical severity. CILD associated with connective tissue disease may be indistinguishable from idiopathic fibrosis, but the former is generally less severe and may respond well to steroids and immunosuppressive therapy.

Pulmonary hypertension

Pulmonary hypertension is defined as elevated pulmonary artery pressure (>25mmHg at rest/30mmHg on exertion)   and can be of primary origin or secondary to the conditions described above e.g. interstitial lung disease or pulmonary emboli. Pulmonary hypertension is seen more frequently with scleroderma, mixed connective tissue disease and rheumatoid arthritis rather than lupus, however, the increased presence of the antiphospholipid syndrome/anti-cardiolipin antibodies in lupus predispose to a thromboembolic aetiology and the incidence of pulmonary hypertension is also increased in the presence of Raynaud's phenomenon.

Symptoms including lethargy, fatigue, angina, syncope and dyspnoea on exertion are relatively non-specific. Diagnosis is, therefore, aided by the presence of distended jugular veins (with prominent a and v waves), right ventricular heave, fixed split S2, hepatomegaly, ascites and peripheral oedema. Investigations should include ECG (changes are consistent with right ventricular hypertrophy) and CXR (cardiomegaly combined with prominent pulmonary arteries can lead to straightening of the left heart border on the background of oligaemic lung fields). Whilst echocardiographic measurement of pulmonary artery pressures may be suggestive, formal diagnosis requires right heart catheterisation which may be accompanied by vasodilator challenge.

Treatment requires specialist supervision and often includes control of any underlying activity of interstitial lung disease with steroids and cytotoxic agents, combined with vasodilators. Prognosis is generally poor but is improved in secondary pulmonary hypertension if an underlying cause can be identified and reversed.

Shrinking lung syndrome (SLS)

Initial lung function measurement in patients with lupus showed that 30% had unexplained shortness of breath with lung volume restriction and sluggish, raised diaphragms. Hence, in 1965 Hoffbran & Beck proposed the "Shrinking Lung" syndrome. Pathophysiology of this disease is still poorly understood and possibly relates to respiratory muscle weakness (predominantly the diaphragm), caused by an unknown myopathic process without documented abnormality of other lung tissue. There is, however, insufficient evidence to support this.

SLS should be considered when lupus patients present with unexplained dyspnoea or chest pain in the presence of reduced lung fields but this diagnosis is thought to be rare and remains a diagnosis of exclusion.

Dr Richard W Lee
Academic Clinical Fellow
   Allergy & Respiratory Medicine
Guy's and St Thomas' Hospitals
London

Prof Kevin A Davies
Professor of Medicine & Honorary
   Consultant Rheumatologist
Brighton & Sussex Medical School
University of Sussex
Brighton
East Sussex BN1 9PX

The Kidneys and Lupus

Introduction

The overall survival of patients with lupus nephritis has improved considerably over the last few decades; from less than 50 % survival at 5 years in the 1960s to over 80% survival at 20 years in the 1990s. This improved survival is due to a combination of factors: including the wider use of corticosteroids and immuno-suppressants and the availability of more effective anti-hypertensive drugs, antibiotics, renal dialysis and transplantation. Early deaths from extra-renal lupus and infection are now uncommon but, instead, renal failure and cardiovascular disease have emerged as important determinants of morbidity and mortality.

Pathogenesis

The pathogenesis of lupus in general, and lupus nephritis in particular, is complex and multifactorial.
See chapter - Genetics

Clinical phenotypes

The American College of Rheumatology has published criteria for the classification of the disease.
See - Diagnosis of Lupus - Specific Symptoms

In many patients, lupus is characterised by intermittent flares of constitutional symptoms, without evidence of major organ involvement. Involvement of major organ systems may occur in the heart, lungs, kidneys or central nervous system (Table 1). These are responsible for most of the mortality and morbidity in this disorder. These manifestations may develop asynchronously over time and this can lead to delays in establishing the diagnosis.

Lupus Nephritis

Clinically apparent nephritis develops in about 40-75 % of patients with lupus and the kidney is the organ most commonly affected. The diagnosis is made by the presence of proteinuria plus or minus haematuria. All patients with lupus should have their urine tested for protein and blood at each clinic visit. Nephritis typically develops early in the course of lupus and, in most patients, lupus nephritis will have appeared within 5 years of diagnosis.

Three major patterns of lupus nephritis have been defined, based on renal histology: focal proliferative, diffuse proliferative and membranous glomerulonephritis. This classification has subsequently been expanded by a World Health Organisation (WHO) committee (Table 2). Patients with minimal changes or mesangial glomerulonephritis (WHO class I and II lesions) usually have an inherently low rate of progressive renal failure. Patients with membranous nephropathy (WHO class V) have an intermediate prognosis for renal function. By contrast, patients with focal or diffuse proliferative glomerulonephritis (WHO class III and IV) have a high risk of progressive renal failure. This classification was revised in 2003 by the International Society of Nephrology and the Renal Pathology Society. The histological classes range from normal by light microscopy (class I) to advanced sclerotic nephritis (class VI).

Renal Presentation

In almost all cases, lupus nephritis develops in patients with evident systemic lupus erythematosus and extra-renal symptoms such as a rash, arthralgia, Raynaud's phenomenon and pleuro-pericarditis predominate. Rarely, renal disease may be the presenting feature of lupus with a small number of patients subsequently, after a period of months to years, developing extra-renal signs of lupus.

Proteinuria is a common finding and is often accompanied by a nephrotic syndrome. This is usually accompanied by various degrees of impairment of renal function. Microscopic haematuria is common but an acute nephritic syndrome is not. A few patients present with a rapidly progressive glomerulonephritis which may be severe enough to lead to acute renal failure. In such patients, a diffuse crescentic nephritis with intra-capillary glomerular thrombi is often seen.

Investigations in Lupus (Table 3)

Laboratory tests

Patients with active lupus commonly have a leucopenia, lymphopenia and thrombocytopenia, often in association with an anaemia of the normochromic normocytic type. The anaemia may result from immune-mediated haemolysis with a positive Coombs' test. An elevated serum creatinine concentration indicates underlying renal involvement, this is an adverse prognostic factor predicting subsequent development of renal failure. The presence of haematuria and proteinuria, particularly if accompanied by active urinary sediment with red cells and casts, is suggestive of active renal disease.

Patients with lupus, in common with those with other autoimmune rheumatic diseases, have raised polyclonal immunoglobulin concentrations but a normal acute phase response providing there is no additional infection. The erythrocyte sedimentation rate (ESR), which is affected by serum proteins and acute phase reactants, has come to be regarded as unreliable in diagnosis. It can, however, be a useful non-specific marker for distinguishing between active and inactive lupus. It may be normal even in the presence of major organ involvement and, conversely, may remain raised in remission. C reactive protein, the classical acute phase protein, is seldom raised in active disease unless the exacerbation is accompanied by serositis or infection. Neither the ESR nor CRP is specific for active lupus so their usefulness in monitoring disease activity has to be interpreted in this light.

Immunology

Patients with lupus almost invariably express antibodies to components of the cell nucleus (ANA). A fluorescent antinuclear test is positive in greater than 95% of patients. In this test, various staining patterns (homogeneous, speckled, rim, nucleolar) can be demonstrated depending on the content of different autoantibodies in the serum. A positive fluorescent ANA test is useful because of its sensitivity, although it lacks specificity and a positive fluorescent ANA test can be found in other connective tissue diseases. More specific, but less sensitive, findings include anti-double-stranded DNA (anti-dsDNA) and anti-Sm autoantibodies. Anti-dsDNA antibodies bind the helical backbone of native DNA, whereas anti-Sm antibodies bind to proteins on an RNA-protein complex termed snRNP. Antibodies to double stranded DNA have the highest specificity for SLE but are only present in about 50% of patients with lupus. The interpretation of anti-dsDNA antibodies is also complicated by the lack of standardisation and various assays for anti-DNA antibodies are currently available: the most commonly used are the ELISA, Crithidia immunofluorescence assay and the Farr radiobinding assay. These assays differ in the source of DNA and the physical chemical properties of the anti-dsDNA antibodies detected. In general, anti-dsDNA antibody levels reflect disease activity, particularly if accompanied by falling complement levels. Antinuclear and anti-dsDNA antibody levels have been less consistently related to features of active glomerulonephritis.

Patients with lupus will often have a false positive response to serological tests for syphilis such as the Venereal Disease Research Laboratory (VDRL) and rapid plasma reagin (RPR) tests because of antibodies to cardiolipin or other phospholipids. Often, antibodies to phospholipids will also interfere with clotting tests resulting in prolongation of the partial thromboplastin time. Anti-cardiolipin antibodies and/or the lupus anticoagulant are also found in patients with the anti-phospholipid syndrome and are associated with arterial thrombosis and miscarriages.

Reduced serum complement concentrations are useful in diagnosis and in assessing disease activity. Many patients with lupus have activation of the complement cascade with consumption of C1q, C4 and C3. Persistent C3 or CH_{50} complement depression has been associated with progression of renal disease in some patients.

Although changes in laboratory tests are extremely useful indicators of disease activity, most doctors do not base therapeutic decisions solely upon them because their sensitivity is less than absolute. Disease activity assessment in lupus must use the additional information provided by the clinical features.

Role of renal biopsy

A renal biopsy is justified when there is evidence of glomerular disease, particularly if this is accompanied by extra-renal features of disease. Glomerular disease is likely if there is proteinuria (>200mg/24 hour; or protein/creatinine ratio >100mg/mmol), and/or haematuria (>10 dysmorphic red blood cells per high power field, or casts of red and white blood cells), with or without renal insufficiency. Histology allows an assessment of disease activity and provides a basis for therapeutic options as well as providing prognostic information.

Monitoring disease activity

Disease monitoring should always include an assessment of clinical symptoms. Objective laboratory measurements of anaemia, thrombocytopenia, leucopenia, lymphopenia, serum creatinine and estimated glomerular filtration rate (modification of diet in renal failure (MDRD) equation) is useful for monitoring lupus activity. The levels of complement and auto-antibodies, including antinuclear antibodies, anti-dsDNA antibodies may be useful markers of disease activity. Urinalysis should be performed at each visit. The persistence/emergence of haematuria and/or proteinuria suggests active renal disease.

Approach to the therapy of lupus treatment

The majority of patients with lupus are successfully managed with non-steroidal anti-inflammatory agents, hydroxychloroquine and low dose corticosteroids. Drug regimens are increased in response to flares and gradually tapered during periods of remission. High dose corticosteroids and immunosuppressive drugs are reserved for patients with life threatening manifestations including severe lupus nephritis, central nervous system, cardiopulmonary disease or haematological abnormalities such as thrombocytopenia.

Treatment of lupus nephritis

There are several considerations in the approach to the treatment of patients with lupus nephritis. The first is based on the histological severity of the renal lesion. The second is based on the severity of the clinical presentation. The third consideration is the choice of therapy for inducing remission of acute disease and for maintaining remission and treating relapses. The heterogeneity of the clinical course of lupus nephritis and the relatively few randomized controlled trials make choice of treatment difficult and there is still substantial disagreement on the optimum treatment of lupus nephritis.

Mesangial Proliferative Glomerulonephritis (WHO class II)

Most such patients present with proteinuria and microscopic haematuria, often with little in the way of renal impairment. There are no controlled trials to guide treatment. Patients are treated with corticosteroids (0.1-0.5mg/kg prednisolone/day tapering over months) in the hope that this will prevent progression to a more severe glomerulonephritis although this cannot be assured.

Membranous Nephropathy (WHO class V)

In patients with lupus nephritis, the frequency of membranous nephropathy is approximately 12% when the definition of the renal histology is confined to pure membranous nephropathy or with mild mesangial hypercellularity, expansion and scattered deposits (WHO classes Va and Vb). The frequency increases to approximately 26% when there is in addition a focal segmental proliferative (WHO class Vc) or diffuse proliferative glomerulonephritis (WHO class Vd). The clinical presentation is with proteinuria and, in about 50% of cases, a nephrotic syndrome. Patients with WHO class Va and Vb lesions have a low rate of progressive renal failure whilst patients with a WHO class Vc or Vd lesions have higher risk of progressive renal failure which is comparable to that of patients with a proliferative glomerulonephritis. Here, again, there are no controlled trials of treatment and so there is no consensus on treatment. In some studies, patients with WHO class Va and Vb have been treated with prednisolone and a smaller proportion also received methylprednisolone pulses and oral cyclophosphamide or azathioprine. By contrast, most patients with WHO class Vc and Vd have been treated with cyclophosphamide or azathioprine in addition to prednisolone. With these approaches to treatment, the 10-year survival free of death and renal failure in WHO class Va and Vb was 72-92% and in WHO class Vc and Vd was 35-81%. It seems reasonable to treat patients with membranous nephropathy and proliferative glomerulonephritis with cyclophosphamide as well as prednisolone because of the proven efficacy of this regime in patients with proliferative lupus glomerulonephritis. Patients with pure lupus membranous nephropathy with or without minor mesangial proliferation may be treated with prednisolone and consideration should be given to adding in azathioprine, cyclosporin or mycophenolate mofetil as a corticosteroid-sparing agent.

Focal and Diffuse Lupus Proliferative Glomerulonephritis (WHO class III and IV)

As the prognosis of patients with these types of lupus nephritis was much poorer than those of patients with mesangial proliferative glomerulonephritis and membranous nephropathy, these patients have been the focus of most of the clinical trials of treatment. In patients with severe focal proliferative or diffuse proliferative glomerulonephritis, corticosteroids alone will reduce the extra-renal manifestations but are less efficient at preserving renal function. There is now good evidence that the addition of cyclophosphamide to prednisolone confers benefit when compared with patients treated with prednisolone alone. The evidence that azathioprine confers such benefit is less good although this agent may have a role in maintaining remission.

A meta-analysis of randomised controlled studies has shown that when compared with prednisolone on its own, cyclophosphamide and prednisolone reduced the risk of doubling of the serum creatinine (RR 0.59; 95%CI 0.4-0.88) whilst azathioprine did not (RR 0.98; 95% CI 0.36-2.68). Neither drug reduced the risk of developing end stage renal failure although further meta-analysis shows that cyclophosphamide does so. Azathioprine reduced the risk of death (RR 0.60; 95% CI 0.36-0.99) whilst cyclophosphamide did not (RR 0.98; 95%CI 0.53-1.82). Cyclophosphamide increased the risk of sustained amenorrhoea (RR 2.18; 95%CI: 1.10-4.34).

A series of clinical trials from the National Institutes of Health (NIH) provided evidence of the effectiveness of intermittent intravenous cyclophosphamide together with oral prednisolone in preserving renal function in patients with severe lupus nephritis. This regime is preferable to continuous oral cyclophosphamide as it typically leads to a lower cumulative dose of cyclophosphamide. From the NIH data, monthly pulse cyclophosphamide (0.5- 1.0 g/m2) adjusted for the glomerular filtration rate and leucocyte count at 10-14 days is given monthly for the first 6 months, then quarterly for 18-24 months. The longer course of cyclophosphamide has been associated with fewer relapses than a shorter 6 month course but is associated with greater gonadal toxicity. Preliminary data with pulse oral cyclophosphamide has shown encouraging results and, if validated, will minimize the inconvenience associated with intravenous therapy. To reduce the bladder toxicity of intravenous cyclophosphamide, patients should be hydrated either with oral or intravenous fluid and 2-mercaptoethane sulfonate sodium (mesna) given concomitantly. Prednisolone is given in conjunction with the cyclophosphamide at an initial dose of (0.5-1 mg/Kg/day) for 6-8 weeks with gradual tapering to minimize toxicity. This regime has been reported in detail and checks must be made prior to the use of such immunosuppressive regime.

The clinical benefit of mycophenolate was first confirmed in a number of small uncontrolled studies and then by larger randomized controlled trials. A conclusion from these studies may be that mycophenolate is probably as effective as and less toxic than cyclophosphamide in patients with new onset mild to moderate lupus nephritis.

Another study assessed the role of mycophenolate, azathioprine and quarterly intravenous cyclophosphamide as maintenance therapy in three groups of lupus nephritis patients (mainly classes III and IV) who all received induction with monthly intravenous cyclophosphamide. The cumulative probability of remaining relapse free was higher in the mycophenolate (78%) and azathioprine (58%) compared to the cyclophosphamide group (43%) after a median treatment duration of 29, 30 and 25 months. The event-free survival rates for the composite end-points of death and chronic renal failure were higher in the mycophenolate and azathioprine groups than the cyclophosphamide group.

Hospitalisation, amenorrhoea and infections were lower in the mycophenolate or azathioprine groups, compared to cyclophosphamide.

In summary, further large adequately powered randomised controlled trials and longer term follow up is necessary to establish the role of mycophenolate in induction treatment of lupus nephritis and also as a maintenance therapy.

Drug toxicities

The various drugs used in the treatment of lupus are discussed elsewhere in this book
See chapter - Drug Therapy of Lupus

These additional notes are applicable to lupus nephritis.

Mycophenolate

Mycophenolate is widely used in the field of human organ transplantation. The active metabolite of mycophenolate is an inhibitor of purine synthesis. It blocks the proliferation of activated T and B lymphocytes and decreases antibody formation. Mycophenolate is teratogenic in animal studies and is, therefore, contraindicated during pregnancy. In general, mycophenolate is well tolerated and most of the adverse events respond to a reduction in dose. Gastrointestinal intolerance, particularly nausea and mild to moderate diarrhoea, occur in up to 10-40% of patients. There is an increased risk of infection which can be associated with leucopenia and lymphopenia.

Other therapeutic options
General measures

As with other proteinuric renal diseases, angiotensin converting enzyme inhibitors or angiotensin II receptor blockers are recommended in patients with lupus nephritis. Hyperlipidaemia should be treated with statins in view of the increased risk of vascular disease in patients with lupus. Finally, bone protection in the form of calcium and vitamin D supplements in patients on long term steroids should be used. Biphosphonates are contraindicated in women of childbearing age and these drugs should be avoided in female patients with lupus.

Plasmapheresis

Several studies have examined the role of plasmapheresis in the treatment of patients with SLE and lupus nephritis. Although plasmapheresis was well tolerated with few adverse effects, impact on renal function was disappointing. The controlled trials have either shown slight but insignificant benefit, or no benefit of plasmapheresis. Since removal of autoantibodies leads to a compensatory enhanced production of autoantibodies by pathogenic B-cell clones, the concept of synchronizing plasmapheresis with subsequent pulse cyclophosphamide to target proliferating B-cell clones was introduced. Initial studies have shown good remission rates in patients with lupus nephritis, but patient numbers were small and the dose of cyclophosphamide used was high ($1.2-1.4$ g/m^2). The toxicity was too high to recommend this approach.

Intravenous immunoglobulins

Uncontrolled studies have shown a temporary benefit in lupus patients from the infusion of high doses of intravenous immunoglobulin. Currently, the data on the use of intravenous immunoglobulin in the treatment of lupus nephritis is limited and, as such, this treatment cannot be recommended.

Cyclosporin

Several studies have examined the effectiveness of cyclosporin in the treatment of lupus nephritis. None of these studies were controlled and it is difficult to discern whether cyclosporin was of any benefit in lupus nephritis. The nephrotoxicity of cyclosporin is a major problem and, pending randomized controlled studies comparing this drug with other immunosuppressive agents, it cannot be recommended for use in lupus nephritis.

Methotrexate

Methotrexate may be useful as a steroid-sparing agent in lupus with arthritis and serositis, and may have potential benefits in mild nephritis. Methotrexate is, however, renally excreted and cannot be used in patients with renal impairment.

Androgens or anti-estrogen therapy

The observations that lupus is a disease predominantly affecting young women with a tendency to flare during pregnancy or with oral contraceptive administration, suggests that hormonal factors may be determinants of pathogenesis or severity. Attempts in men to control lupus by manipulating estrogen and testosterone levels have had only modest success. Despite *in vitro* data, there is little evidence to support the use of androgens or anti-estrogen in lupus nephritis.

Monoclonal Antibodies

Several studies have examined the use of monoclonal antibody therapy in patients with lupus nephritis. CD5 is a molecule on the surface of T cells and a subpopulation of B cells, and the use of anti-CD5 ricin A chain immuno-conjugate (CD% PLUS) led to an improvement in urine and laboratory parameters in 5 of 8 patients with glomerulonephritis. This approach in clinical practice remains to be validated

Inhibition of co-stimulation

CD40 binding to CD40 ligand is one of the most important co-stimulatory signals on B cells inducing activation and proliferation. The first open-label study focused on 30 patients with lupus nephritis and showed improvement in serology. This study was halted because of unexpected thromboembolic events. A second double-blind placebo controlled trial of 85 patients with mild to moderate lupus failed to show clinical efficacy over placebo.

Alternative co-stimulatory targets in lupus include the CD2 and CTLA4 receptors and their B-cell co-ligands B&-1 and B7-2. The T cell antigen CTLA-4 linked to murine IgGg2a (CTLA4Ig) has been shown to block autoantibody production and prolong life span in NZB/NZW F_1 mice. The immunosuppressive properties of these classes of drugs have not been thoroughly tested, and warrant further testing before any recommendations can be made of their efficacy in lupus nephritis.

Cell-depleting and anti-cytokine therapy

Rituximab is a chimeric monoclonal antibody against the B-cell marker CD20 and several open clinical trials suggest that B-cell depletion with rituximab can improve clinical manifestations of lupus. However, some patients developed elevated human anti-chimeric antibodies. When a combination of rituximab, high dose steroids and cyclophosphamide was used in lupus 20 out of 21 patients experienced effective B-cell depletion, with 9 patients remaining off immunosuppressive therapy at a follow-up of 12-46 months. In another report, 9 patients with class III and IV nephritis treated with rituximab and steroids also described good efficacy, with partial remission in 80% and complete remission in 50% (30%). These encouraging results need to be confirmed by randomized controlled studies.

Oral tolerance therapy

Oral tolerance therapy may have a role in the treatment of lupus if the offending antigens can be identified. A phase III trial of 317 randomised patients has been completed using the B-cell tolerogen LJP394. Preliminary results indicate a sustained reduction in anti-dsDNA antibodies and improvement in health-related quality of life. Additional studies are on- going.

Immune ablation and stem cell transplantation

Procedure-related mortality varies among studies between 5 and 12%. The exact role of autologous stem cell transplant using high-dose cyclophosphamide for lupus has not yet been determined and cannot be recommended.

Other newer modalities

Other potential treatments for lupus nephritis include neutralizing antibodies to anti-C5 complement, anti-BAFF (B cell activation factor), a chemokine receptor CCR1 antagonist and human recombinant DNase. These are in the preliminary stages of development.

Prognostic factors in lupus nephritis

Knowledge about prognosis assists physicians in their choice of treatment and provides patients with information on the possible outcomes. Patients with proliferative glomerulonephritis (WHO III and IV) tend to have a worse outcome for renal function when compared to patients with milder lesions. The combination of severe active and chronic histological changes on a renal biopsy is also reported to adversely affect outcome. Patients without chronic histological changes, even in the face of active lupus nephritis, had a lower risk of developing renal failure with 90 % or more remaining free of renal failure after 10 years. A number of clinical variables are associated with a greater probability of renal progression in lupus nephritis. These include: black race, low haematocrit, raised serum creatinine level, presence of hypertension, high urinary protein excretion, low C3 complement and poor socioeconomic status. Failure to respond to prednisolone and cyclophosphamide are also predictors of subsequent development of renal failure, as are nephritic flares.

Dialysis and Transplantation

Between 17-30% of patients with lupus nephritis develop end stage renal failure by 10 years. Both haemodialysis and continuous ambulatory peritoneal dialysis are well tolerated and there is tendency for lupus disease activity to diminish after the start of dialysis. If there is no overt disease activity, immunosuppressants in patients on dialysis may be discontinued and a small dose of prednisolone continued. Overall survival on dialysis is good with a 75% survival at 10 years. Graft survival and function in patients with lupus after transplantation are comparable to those obtained in patients with other diseases and recurrence of lupus nephritis is uncommon after transplantation.

Conclusion

Any patient with symptoms of organic dysfunction (Table 1), supported by laboratory evidence of dysfunction, must be referred to a specialist so that the diagnosis can be established, disease severity assessed and a management plan formulated. Immunosuppressive therapy and corticosteroids have, undoubtedly, had an impact on renal preservation in patients with severe lupus nephritis. No consensus has yet been reached on a number of therapeutic issues including: the optimal induction drug regimen, optimal regimen for treating relapse and maintenance therapy to prevent relapses. However, it is hoped that early diagnosis and treatment will prevent progression of renal damage, which can develop rapidly in those with severe lupus nephritis.

Complications of drug treatment account for much of the morbidity that develops in lupus, in particular, complications of high dose or chronic corticosteroids (infection, osteonecrosis, osteoporosis, coronary artery disease) and cyclophosphamide (infection, sterility, bladder toxicity and malignancy). It is encouraging that mycophenolate has a less toxic side-effect profile than cyclophosphamide. The risk of infections is also substantial in patients taking corticosteroids and immunosuppressants. Infections should be treated with appropriate antibiotics and immunosuppressants will need to be temporarily withdrawn if there is overwhelming sepsis or neutropenia.

Both the hospital physicians and general practitioners have a very important role to play in the management of these patients, especially in monitoring drug toxicity, blood pressure and renal function. Regular clinical review of the patient's condition, together with laboratory tests and urinalysis to detect marrow depression, disease activity or progressive disease is mandatory in the management of these patients.

Table 1. Major organ involvement in Lupus

Renal
Mesangial, focal, and diffuse proliferative glomerulonephritis
Membranous nephropathy
Glomerulosclerosis
Tubulointerstitial nephritis

Neurologic/psychiatric
Diffuse neurologic syndromes (organic brain syndromes, psychosis, affective disorders, meningitis)
Focal neurologic syndromes (seizures, cerebrovascular events, transverse myelitis)
Movement disorders (chorea, cerebellar ataxia, Parkinson-like)
Peripheral neuropathy (symmetric sensorimotor, mononeuritis multiplex, Guillain-Barré)

Pulmonary
Parenchymal disorders (pneumonitis, alveolar haemorrhage, bronchiolitis obliterans)
Vascular (pulmonary hypertension, pulmonary embolism)
Shrinking lung syndrome

Cardiac
Myocarditis
Endocarditis
Coronary vasculitis

Gastrointestinal
Mesenteric vasculitis
Inflammatory bowel disease
Pancreatitis

Table 2. The World Health Organisation Classification of Lupus Nephritis

Class I: Normal or minimal change disease (1%-4%)
           (a) Nil (by all techniques)
           (b) Normal by light microscopy but deposits by electron
               or immunofluorescence microscopy

Class II: Mesangial glomerulonephritis (20%)
           (a) Mesangial widening and/or mild hypercellularity
           (b) Moderate hypercellularity

Class III: Focal proliferative glomerulonephritis (25%)
           (a) "Active" necrotizing lesions
           (b) "Active and sclerosing lesions"
           (c) Sclerosing lesions

Class IV: Diffuse proliferative glomerulonephritis (37%)
           (a) Without segmental lesions
           (b) With "active" necrotising lesions
           (c) With "active" and sclerosing lesions
           (d) With sclerosing lesions

Class V: Membranous glomerulonephritis (13%)
           (a) Pure membranous glomerulonephritis
           (b) Associated with lesions of category II (a or b)
           (c) Associated with lesions of category III (a - c)*
           (d) Associated with lesions of category IV (a - d)*

*Alternatively, cases in these subcategories may be classified under category IV

Table 3. Investigations in Systemic Lupus Erythematosus

Full blood examination
  anaemia, cytopenia

Erythrocyte sedimentation rate
  Long half life
  Non-specific and may not mirror disease activity
  Frequently elevated during active SLE

C-reactive protein level
  Raised levels are suggestive of superimposed infection

Complements, C3 and C4
  Levels are decreased in active disease

Autoantibodies
  anti-dsDNA
  antinuclear antibody
  anti-Sm
  anti-histone (in drug-induced SLE)
  anti-Ro and anti-La (also in Sjögren's syndrome)

Tests of renal function
  Urea, electrolytes and creatinine levels
  24-hour urine protein level
  Urine microscopy
  Renal biopsy

Cardiac and pulmonary investigations, if evidence of involvement

Dr Wai Y Tse
Consultant Physician and Honorary Senior Lecturer
Department of Nephrology
Derriford Hospital
Derriford Road
Plymouth PL6 8DH

Dr Dwomoa Adu
Consultant Physician
Department of Nephrology
Queen Elizabeth Hospital
Edgbaston
Birmingham B15 2TH

Central Nervous System Involvement in Lupus and Antiphospholipid (Hughes) Syndrome

Introduction

Central nervous system (CNS) involvement has been emphasised as one of the major lupus manifestations since the first descriptions of the disease and is among the leading causes of morbidity and mortality. Its recognition and treatment continue to represent a major diagnostic and therapeutic challenge. Conventional tests give the prevalence of neurological abnormalities in lupus as 40-50%. However, with the recognition of the antiphospholipid syndrome (APS) and its striking array of neurological manifestations and the more penetrating studies of neuropsychiatric and cognitive changes in lupus, this percentage might become higher.

Clinical Manifestations

The spectrum of CNS involvement is wide and encompasses almost the whole spectrum of neurological diseases (Table 1). By far the most frequent manifestations are headache, depression, psychiatric illness ranging from mild affective disorder to full blown psychosis and generalised seizures. The neuropsychiatric events are unpredictable and can occur at any time in the course of the disease, occasionally even preceding the onset of systemic disease. A neurological disorder may occur as an isolated event or in association with other signs of systemic disease activity. Multiple neurological events may occur together.

Headaches are a very common complaint in lupus. They may be migrainous and last for days or weeks. The headaches are often intractable, unresponsive to narcotic analgesics and can antedate the diagnosis by many years. Epilepsy is an important complication of lupus patients and can present as generalised "grand mal", focal, temporal lobe or "petit mal". Seizures can be a primary event resulting from the direct effect of active lupus on the CNS, or may also occur as a consequence of infection or metabolic abnormality. Ten per cent of lupus patients develop seizures and a strong association between the presence of antiphospholipid antibodies (aPL) and seizures is now well established.

Neurocognitive dysfunction is also a common feature in lupus and may be present in up to 80% of the patients with active CNS manifestations and in 40% of overall lupus patients. The various studies of cognitive function suggest considerable diversity in the type of cognitive impairment, including attention and concentration, various aspects of verbal and non-verbal memory including working memory, verbal fluency, visuo-spatial skills, psychomotor speed and cognitive flexibility.

Psychosis, depression and anxiety are the most frequently cited psychiatric disorders in lupus, although both frequency and pathophysiological relationship to the disease remain controversial.

Vasculopathy due to thrombotic events in the presence of aPL is a well known cause of ischemic cerebral disease. Often the features (as well as the MRI lesions) are widespread and frequently mis-diagnosed as "vasculitis". Several cases of focal neurologic manifestations associated with aPL in lupus patients have been reported. These include cerebral vein thrombosis and chorea. Thrombosis of microvessels in the retina and the inner ear causing amaurosis fugax, blindness and sensorineural hearing loss, respectively, are features associated with the presence of aPL.

Transverse myelitis is a rare manifestation of lupus, estimated as less than 1% of complications. The presentation of acute transverse myelopathy usually occurs early in the course of lupus. Serologic parameters of disease activity are not always remarkable. MRI or CT/Myelogram should be performed to exclude any cord compression requiring surgery. Neurogenic bladder may persist despite motor recovery. There is a strong association between transverse myelitis and the presence of aPL.

Less common in lupus than in primary vasculitis, peripheral neuropathy may present as sensory polyneuropathy (stocking-glove distribution), mononeuritis multiplex and mixed motor and sensory polyneuropathy, while ocular motor abnormalities, facial palsy and trigeminal neuropathy, may be presenting symptoms of cranial neuropathies. Acute ascending motor paralysis, indistinguishable from Guillain-Barre, narcolepsy, aseptic meningitis, pseudotumour cerebri, normal pressure hydrocephalus and myasthenia gravis are many of the rare CNS manifestations described in patients with lupus.

Diagnosis

The diagnosis of CNS lupus is primarily clinical and follows exclusion of other possible causes such as sepsis, drug effects (steroids), metabolic disturbances (uraemia) and severe hypertension. Evidence of active disease in other organs is helpful but not always present. There is no single test that is diagnostic. A careful history and physical examination coupled with routine laboratory studies (including coagulation) may help distinguish CNS lupus from neuropsychiatric dysfunction due to other causes. CSF examination has proved disappointing, apart from its use in the exclusion of infection. Elevated CSF IgG, IgM or IgA and the presence of oligoclonal bands have been observed in CNS lupus.

Neuroimaging

Imaging tools may aid in the diagnosis of CNS lupus. However, despite many different types of neuroimaging test abnormalities described in CNS lupus, there is no specific finding that is diagnostic. Indeed, the heterogeneous nature of the disease could explain the inconsistent association between clinical symptoms and neuroimaging studies.

The MRI has been shown to be superior to CT scanning in detecting lesions in CNS lupus. However, the finding of focal lesions on brain MRI must be interpreted with caution. Previous studies have reported that a few asymptomatic lupus patients without a history of CNS disease will show focal white matter lesions. This is more likely to occur in patients with aPL, hypertension or other cardiovascular risk factors.

Single-photon emission computed tomography (SPECT) uses tomographic reconstruction of single photons emitted by radio-labelled tracer for the determination of cerebral blood flow. Abnormal SPECT scans are frequently observed in subjects with focal and diffuse CNS lupus and in children with lupus in whom the diagnosis is especially difficult to document. In general, SPECT scans have shown a high sensitivity (90%) but low specificity (30%) in CNS lupus patients. Clearly, non-lupus causes of CNS disturbances can result in an abnormal SPECT scan. Conversely, a normal SPECT scan may provide evidence against active CNS lupus.

Positron emission tomography (PET) is a radionuclide technique that uses unstable isotopes for measuring cerebral glucose uptake or consumption, cerebral oxygen uptake or blood flow. PET has been found to show abnormalities in milder CNS disorder, such as cognitive dysfunction, which do not show up in MRI.

Other manifestations of lupus neuroimaging include cerebral atrophy, venous thrombosis, venous infarction and intracranial calcification. Sulcal enlargement with or without ventricular enlargement is common in CNS lupus and seems related to disease duration and long term steroid therapy, rather than an intrinsic manifestation of CNS lupus.

Treatment

Due to the lack of controlled randomised trials, there is a desperate need to assess the efficacy of various therapeutic interventions in CNS lupus, where the treatment is still empirical and based on clinical experience.

Focal CNS Manifestations

One of the most important advances in the treatment of CNS lupus has come from the recognition of the APS and the importance of thrombotic mechanisms in the development of a number of CNS manifestations in lupus patients. The presence of aPL is strongly associated with thrombotic CNS events. The most common manifestations of focal CNS disease in lupus patients are transient ischemic attacks and ischemic stroke. Many lupus patients with cerebral ischemia and aPL, who would have previously received high dose of corticosteroids and/or immunosuppression, are today being successfully treated with anticoagulation. Immunosuppression should only be used in patients with active lupus disease. There is no evidence so far to support its use in patients with APS. Minimum treatment requires antiaggregant therapy as a prophylactic measure, but long-term anticoagulation with warfarin is mandatory in patients with APS-associated stroke. Other focal CNS manifestations, such as demyelinating syndrome, transverse myelitis, chorea, migraine and seizures, when associated with aPL, may also benefit from anticoagulation.

Severe diffuse CNS manifestations

Acute confusional state, generalized seizures, major depression and psychosis, and severe cognitive dysfunction generally require corticosteroids in the first instance. High dose of corticosteroids may only be used in severe cases and preferably for short terms. Pulse intravenous cyclophosphamide therapy may help when more severe manifestations are refractory to corticosteroids and other immunosuppressive agents. Plasmapheresis, IVIG, intrathecal methotrexate and dexamethasone, mycophenolate mofetil and rituximab deserve further studies to confirm their usefulness in the treatment of CNS lupus.

Table 1. Major neuropsychiatric syndromes in Systemic Lupus Erythematosus

- Headaches
- Focal and generalised seizures
- Ischemic cerebrovascular accidents
- Organic brain syndrome (delirium, cognitive impairment, impaired memory or concentration)
- Psychiatric disorders (psychosis, depression, phobias, schizophrenia, catatonia)
- Peripheral neuropathy (radiculopathy, plexopathy, mononeuritis, polyneuropathy, autonomic neuropathy)
- Transverse myelitis
- Movement disorders (particularly chorea)
- Myasthenia gravis

Dr Munther A Khamashta
Senior Lecturer/Consultant Physician
Director, Lupus Research Unit
St Thomas' Hospital
London SE1 7EH

Mood Disorders and Lupus

Defining mood disorders

Mood disorders include depression and generalised anxiety and are one of the most frequently experienced type of psychological problem for people with lupus. Other common neuropsychiatric manifestations of lupus such as cognitive impairment, epilepsy, psychosis and catatonia are outlined elsewhere.

See chapters - CNS Involvement in Lupus and Antiphospholipid (Hughes) Syndrome.

It is important to establish diagnostic criteria for mood disorders before it is possible to plan effective strategies to enable people with these conditions to make sustainable improvements in their mood.

An effective initial screening method (prior to appointments) can make use of a retrospective questionnaire assessment such as Zigmond and Snaith's 14-symptom Hospital Anxiety and Depression Scale, which takes little time to complete. This provides information on how severe these symptoms are but is not a diagnostic tool *per se*. Simple mood diaries are an effective way of self-monitoring daily mood; these can be completed as frequently as the person wishes (e.g. three times a day) and giving as much or little detail as they want (e.g. a single numerical rating on a 0-10 scale and/or free narrative).

The terms *depressed* and *anxious* have been assimilated into everyday language but the mood disorders these symptoms reflect are based on clear medical diagnoses. Whilst these may be the most salient term for a person experiencing an acute episode of mood disturbance, health professionals must listen to the mood symptoms their patients are describing and map these along the parallel continuums from happiness and calmness to enduring sadness or generalised anxiety. However, people with lupus are rarely at the extreme ends of the continuum and will often report moderately depressed or anxious mood states and judgment is required to determine if these require help.

An episode of major depression is classified by the American Psychiatric Association's Diagnostic and Statistical Manual (DSM) as a period of at least 2 weeks of having depressed mood or lack of interest in activities and anhedonia (the lack of pleasure from previously enjoyed activities). These problems should be experienced most of the day and every day for this period. In addition to this, classification requires the individual to have four or more of the following associated problems:

- Change in appetite or change in weight
- Hypersomnia or insomnia (especially waking early)

- Restlessness or feeling slowed down
- Fatigue or loss of energy
- Guilt and feelings of worthlessness
- Inability to concentrate or indecisiveness
- Suicidal ideation

The World Health Organization's International Statistical Classification of Diseases and Related Health Problems (ICD) section on mental and behavioural disorders codes depressive episodes as mild, moderate or severe (F32.0, F32.1 and F32.2, respectively). All three codes are outlined as sharing the features of depressed mood, loss of interest and enjoyment and reduced energy levels leading to diminished activity due to increased fatigability after only slight effort is common. Other common symptoms are reduced concentration and attention, reduced self-esteem and self-confidence, ideas of guilt and unworthiness, bleak and pessimistic views of the future, ideas or acts of self-harm or suicide, disturbed sleep and diminished appetite. For all three severity grades of depressed mood it is stated that a duration of at least 2 weeks is usually required for diagnosis unless the onset is rapid and severe.

The symptoms within both of these sets of diagnostic criteria have to be seen in the context of the disease process where a person with lupus might experience sleep disturbance and diminished appetite, especially within a flare. There is some potential for overlap with fatigue and disability from lupus, but the criterion of feeling slowed down might be best interpreted and explained as referring to a cognitive experience rather than as physical problems. These symptoms are defined as 'somatic' in the ICD and consideration of these will help avoid 'false positive' diagnoses. It is assumed that these criteria are being applied to individuals who have already received a diagnosis of lupus. Research indicates that people with lupus in their early journey to obtaining the diagnosis, when symptoms may fluctuate and objective tests prove inconclusive, can be wrongly misdiagnosed with a mood disorder and this may impact on satisfaction with healthcare interactions in the future.

A less intense but prolonged version of depression is called dysthymic disorder or minor depression; this is classified as depressed mood most of the day, more days than not for at least 2 years in the DSM, and very similarly in the ICD where it is not so strictly defined (code F34.1). This will probably be the most common type of depressed mood that will be seen in a clinical practice.

Generalised anxiety disorder is distinct from phobias and pure obsessive thought disorders and can be classified in a very similar way to depression. The DSM classifies this using the criteria of excessive, uncontrollable worry about several events (which could include one's state of health) more days than not for a period of at least 6 months that has an impact on social functioning or work ability. In addition to this, to be classified the individual is required to have four or more of the following associated problems:

- Feeling restless or 'edgy'
- Experiencing fatigue easily
- Having difficulty concentrating
- Being irritable without reason
- Experiencing muscle tension (particularly of the shoulders/neck)
- Having disturbed sleep (especially onset insomnia)

The criterion of muscle tension may be experienced in rheumatic disease. It is also clear that (major) depression and (generalised) anxiety have a large overlap in content of their listed symptom and associated thought processes. This will, hopefully, be clarified in the forthcoming revision to the DSM criteria, which are being redeveloped. The ICD already defines concomitant anxiety and depressive disorder (code F41.2). Fortunately, both conditions can be tackled by similar medical treatments and psychological therapies.

Given that there are problems with accurate recall of psychological processes, the criteria for depression and anxiety ideally require some form of daily mood assessment. There are many good measures of mood available; two classic measures are Watson and colleagues' Positive and Negative Affect Schedule and Lorr and McNair's Profile of Mood States. Both of these questionnaires cover depression (versus elation) and anxiety (versus calmness) although it is feasible, and indeed may be preferable, to allow patients to define a diary system for recording aspects of their mood without the formality of such scales.

A further simple method of getting to the heart of the issue of depression (reflecting the above criteria) is the use of two screening questions composed by Arroll and colleagues:

- "During the past month have you often been bothered by feeling down, depressed, or hopeless?"
- "During the past month have you often been bothered by little interest or pleasure in doing things?"

These questions can allow therapeutic skills to be directed to either or both of these issues, as will now be considered further. Alternatively, patients' responses to these questions may be used as the basis for suggesting a referral to local psychological services.

Medications

Antidepressant medications have traditionally been the first-line treatment for mood disorders given the ease of access and known cost-effectiveness. The British National Institute for Health and Clinical Excellence (NICE) currently recommends specific serotonin reuptake inhibitors (SSRIs) over tricyclic antidepressants due to reports of fewer side-effects from the former. However, tricyclics are sometimes given in small doses to reduce muscle tension and thus aid sleep in rheumatic disease, but there is no clear evidence of whether this regimen improves outcomes of mood disorders. Some SSRIs are also suitable for treatment of generalised anxiety. Moreover, people with lupus who also experience fibromyalgia syndrome may well benefit from the improvements in pain and function that certain antidepressants can provide in fibromyalgia.
See chapter - the Joints and Lupus

The Talking Therapies

People with lupus may not be keen to take antidepressants given the number of other medications that they may be taking. NICE suggests offering Cognitive Behavioural Therapy (CBT) for recurrent depression (ICD code F33) when the person is not happy to take antidepressants again. Indeed, NICE recommends psychological therapy over antidepressants as the first option for treatment of new cases of mild to moderate depression; NICE also recommends a combination of antidepressants along with psychological therapy when the case of depression is severe.

The psychological approaches, known collectively as talking therapies, include CBT, Motivational Interviewing, Counselling (from a variety of perspectives i.e. Freudian; Jungian; Humanistic) and Brief Solution-Focused Therapy. The essence of these approaches is to allow people with a mood disorder (or other issue) a safe space to talk over their situation, map out goals about what they want to change and provide them with methods of helping themselves to work towards this change. The application of one of the talking therapies is known to provide improvements in mood for people with lupus if they are willing and able to access such services, particularly if their spouse is also allowed to attend. Local rheumatology departments may have access to a health psychologist or other professional who can deliver a specialised form of talking therapy for people with lupus that may be more able to meet their needs than a general service at the primary care level. In the UK, a health psychologist is someone who specialises in the psychology of physical health, having completed accredited undergraduate, masters and doctoral degree programmes (or equivalent).

'Standards of Care' have been published by the Arthritis and Musculoskeletal Alliance (ARMA) in the UK for a variety of specific rheumatic diseases, including systemic lupus erythematosus. These standards define what evidence-based services and interventions are appropriate for people with lupus and suggest ways of providing them effectively. ARMA propose that CBT-based self-management training should be available for individuals with any rheumatic disease at any stage of their illness via the *Challenging Arthritis* programme run by the charity *Arthritis Care* (for information on local courses see their website) or via the generic Expert Patient Programmes, which are now available throughout the UK within Primary Care Trusts. Cognitive-behavioural approaches can be applied on an individual basis or within *small* group settings (i.e. between 4 and 10 members) and focus upon accessing those cognitions (thought processes), moods and behaviours that lead to depression and anxiety. Many people with lupus will be happy to seek information and learn strategies for self-care through these group-based interventions. However, not all individuals will be able or comfortable with attending such courses. There are computerised CBT interfaces available, one of which (Beating the Blues™) has been approved by NICE and may be an ideal format for people with lupus who want to be flexible about the time, place and level of contact they engage with for psychotherapy to improve their mood.

Summary

Mood disorders, particularly depression and generalised anxiety, are common among people with lupus but there is much that can be done to ameliorate the effects of these conditions. Firstly, it is necessary to actively enquire about people's mood, offer a label for any conditions they describe and discuss whether they wish to receive help. Following this, the sources of help depend on local availability across the modalities described within this chapter.

Ms Elizabeth D Hale
Chartered Health
Psychologist
Dept of Rheumatology
Clinical Research Unit
Russells Hall Hospital
Dudley
West Midlands
DY1 2HQ

Dr Gareth J Treharne
Dept of Psychology
University of Otago
Dunedin
New Zealand

Prof George D Kitas
Consultant
Rheumatologist
Dept of Rheumatology
Clinical Research Unit
Russells Hall Hospital
Dudley
West Midlands
DY1 2HQ

Vasculitis

Introduction

Vasculitis means inflammation of blood vessels. Direct inflammatory changes within the wall of a blood vessel (i.e. vasculitis) frequently causes necrosis to the vessel wall, hence the term often used 'necrotizing vasculitis'.

Vasculitis can either be primary (e.g. polyarteritis nodosa, Wegener's granulomatosis) occurring in the absence of a recognised cause or associated disease, or secondary to an established disease, (e.g. rheumatoid arthritis or systemic lupus erythematosus), or secondary to infection such as hepatitis B, C or HIV.

The consequence of vasculitis depends on the size, site and number of blood vessels involved. The spectrum of involvement ranges from relatively mild disease affecting small vessels or isolated to a single organ, to rapidly life threatening multi-system disease. When muscular arteries are involved they can develop focal or segmental lesions. Focal lesions indicate only part of the wall is involved which may become weak, leading to aneurysm formation which may be followed by rupture. Segmental lesions indicate that the whole circumference of the vessel is involved and is more common and this will lead to narrowing or occlusion with distal infarction. Haemorrhage into, or infarction of, vital internal organs are the most serious complications of vasculitis. Prior to the introduction of cyclophosphamide the mortality of the primary vasculitides, particularly Wegener's granulomatosis and polyarteritis nodosa, was over 80% by one year. Improved treatment has dramatically improved the survival but there is still significant morbidity from the disease (and/or its treatment).

Classification

An understanding of the different types of vasculitis is helped by understanding classification. A number of different classification systems have been used, a favoured system being shown in Table 1 based on the dominant vessels involved and dividing diseases into primary and secondary vasculitis. Lupus is, obviously, included as one of the secondary vasculitides and most commonly is associated with small vessel vasculitis but can involve small vessels and medium arteries when the consequences are much more serious (see below). The importance of this classification is that the different groups require different types of treatment and this is shown in Table 2. Patients with giant cell arteritis, which is the most common vasculitis seen in general practice, are usually treated with high dose corticosteroids and rarely with any other drugs. Patients with classical polyarteritis nodosa which is rare (see below) may be treated with steroids and/or cyclophosphamide but can also respond to anti-viral therapy and plasma exchange. It is the group of diseases which overlap between medium arteries and small vessels, including severe lupus vasculitis, that are the most serious and life-threatening and these usually require treatment with high dose steroids and cyclophosphamide. In contrast, pure small vessel disease which most commonly involves the skin usually responds to relatively low doses of corticosteroids.

Epidemiology

The vasculitides are relatively rare, the most common being giant cell arteritis with an incidence of approximately 1 patient per 10,000 over the age of 50 per year and cutaneous vasculitis with an incidence of approximately 30/million/year. Taking all the other systemic vasculitides together, their incidence is probably in the region of 40/million/year and, specifically looking at lupus associated with severe systemic vasculitis, the incidence is probably less than 5 per million per year. This means that a practice of approximately 10,000 will see one or two patients with giant cell arteritis each year, probably one patient with Wegener's every 10 years and one with severe lupus vasculitis every 10-20 years. The consequence of giant cell arteritis with potential blindness is well known but it is important to recognise the other vasculitides because they are now treatable/curable diseases, having previously had median survival of less than 6 months before the introduction of drugs such as cyclophosphamide.

Clinical features

The clinical presentation of vasculitis varies dependent on the underlying disease. The most important organ involved in primary systemic vasculitis is the kidney. Any patient with suspected vasculitis should have labstix testing of the urine and in the presence of systemic illness haematuria and proteinuria are an important and serious prognostic sign. In those circumstances the differential diagnosis would include infection such as bacterial endocarditis, malignancy, connective tissue disease with or without vasculitis such as lupus and systemic vasculitis, particularly Wegener's granulomatosis, Churg-Strauss syndrome and microscopic polyangiitis.

The most common clinical feature of vasculitis is a skin rash. Particularly common is a nonthrombocytopaenic purpuric rash often affecting the lower limbs. This is the classical presentation of Henoch Schönlein purpura which is much more common in children than in adults but is also a feature of all the other primary vasculitides involving small vessels. Other clinical features depend on the organs involved. In Wegener's granulomatosis there is frequently ENT involvement with nasal crusting and recurrent nose bleeds which can precede the onset of vasculitis by months or years. Similarly, in Churg-Strauss syndrome the early features are those of adult or late onset asthma which can also precede systemic vasculitis by months or years. Asthma associated with a particularly high eosinophil count and the development of a rash should always alert the doctor to consider systemic vasculitis and, again, if this is unrecognised and untreated, it can be fatal due to kidney and also (in Churg-Strauss) heart involvement.

Systemic vasculitis complicating lupus will often present with severe skin rashes which may be necrotic leading to gangrene. Deteriorating renal function is also important and in a patient with lupus with new proteinuria or haematuria a renal biopsy and formal assessment by a nephrologist is essential and urgent. Cerebral symptoms in lupus can also be a consequence of vasculitis as can peripheral neuropathy. Peripheral nerve symptoms can be difficult to detect but sudden onset of numbness or weakness in a patient who is generally unwell should suggest the possibility of vasculitis and is commoner in patients with Churg-Strauss syndrome and lupus than in the other vasculitides.

Investigations

As indicated above, the single most important investigation in a patient with suspected vasculitis is urine testing. In a systemically unwell person the presence of blood and protein in the urine indicates the necessity for urgent referral and probably urgent treatment. Other investigations that can be helpful include a routine blood count and ESR. Anaemia of chronic disease develops quite rapidly in many vasculitides and most are associated with a high acute phase response as shown by a high ESR and/or CRP. Basic tests for renal and liver function are important to detect deteriorating renal function and mild derangement of liver enzymes is common in all inflammatory diseases including vasculitis, however, very high levels might indicate an associated hepatitis, such as hepatitis B or C infection.

Immunological tests are helpful. A low level of complement (C3 and C4) is often a feature of secondary vasculitis due to rheumatoid arthritis, lupus, Sjögren's Syndrome or infection, but is very rarely seen in patients with primary vasculitis. High levels of the appropriate antibodies are seen, for example DNA binding and Sm antibodies, in lupus vasculitis and rheumatoid factor in rheumatoid vasculitis. The primary vasculitides - Wegener's granulomatosis, Churg-Strauss syndrome and microscopic polyangiitis are associated with a relatively new antibody known as ANCA (antineutrophil cytoplasmic antibody). Recent studies have shown that the specificity of this antibody can also help differentiate disease in that when the antibody acts against proteinase 3 it is strongly associated with Wegener's granulomatosis, but ANCA with specificity against other enzymes, particularly myeloperoxidase, is often found in Churg-Strauss syndrome and microscopic polyangiitis.

Investigations otherwise depend on the organ involved. Haemoptysis which is common in Wegener's requires a chest X-ray and nasal crusting or nasal discharge or bleeding indicates a necessity for ENT referral and sinus X-rays. Polyarteritis nodosa is sometimes diagnosed on angiography but this requires specialist referral and in-hospital investigation.

In patients with suspected giant cell arteritis, temporal artery biopsy is often advocated but not always necessary. In any case where the diagnosis is in doubt it is useful to obtain a temporal artery biopsy because a positive biopsy indicates the necessity for long-term treatment with steroids.

Treatment

The introduction of cyclophosphamide has had the most dramatic effect on the treatment of the severe systemic vasculitides and has improved survival to between 80 and 90% at 5 years. Cyclophosphamide may be given continuously in tablet form but is associated with a significant risk of cystitis and some increased risk of late bladder cancer. For some years many patients have been given cyclophosphamide in pulsed form, usually intravenously, and a recent study from Europe has shown that this way of giving cyclophosphamide is equally efficaceous but associated with significantly less side effects. Patients requiring cyclophosphamide need to be monitored carefully, and patients with vasculitis need long-term follow up shared between general practitioner and the hospital because of the risk of relapse and toxicity from their treatment. The role of other immunosuppressive and biologic drugs has been highlighted in the last few years with mycophenolate mofetil proving to be particularly useful for lupus nephritis. This drug may also have a role as an alternative to cyclophosphamide in patients with vasculitis but studies for this are ongoing. There is also a lot of interest in the biologic treatment of vasculitis, particularly rituximab which has been used in many cases of severe relapsing Wegener's granulomatosis and is now a significant advance in treatment of severe lupus, and may be an appropriate treatment to consider where cyclophosphamide causes problems in severe vasculitis complicating lupus.

Conclusion

Recent advances in the understanding of the vasculitides have led to a dramatic improvement in outcome, increased recognition of the different types of vasculitis and an apparent increase in their incidence. Although rare, they are important because they are treatable and should and can be recognised and referred appropriately from primary care.

Table I - Classification of systemic vasculitis

Dominant vessels involved	Primary	Secondary
Large arteries	Giant cell arteritis Takayasu's arteritis Isolated CNS angiitis	Aortitis associated with RA Infection (e.g. syphilis)
Medium arteries	Classical PAN Kawasaki disease	Infection (e.g. hepatitis B)
Small vessels and medium arteries	Wegener's granulomatosis* Churg-Strauss syndrome* Microscopic polyangiitis*	Vasculitis secondary to RA and SLE Sjögren's Syndrome Drugs Infection (e.g. HIV)
Small vessels (leukocytoclastic)	Henoch-Schönlein-purpura Essential mixed cryoglobulinaemia Cutaneous leukocytoclastic angiitis	Drugs† Infection (e.g. hepatitis B & C) Vasculitis secondary to RA and SLE

PAN = Polyarteritis nodosa; RA = rheumatoid arthritis; SLE = systemic lupus erythematosus
* Diseases most commonly associated with ANCA (anti-myeloperoxidase and anti-proteinase 3 antibodies), which have a significant risk of renal involvement and which are most responsive to immunosuppression with cyclophosphamide.
† For example, sulphonamides, penicillins, thiazide diuretics and many others.
Reproduced from Scott and Watts
(1994, British Journal of Rheumatology 33: 897-898)

Table 2 - Relationship between vessel size and response to treatment

Dominant vessel involved	Corticosteroids alone	Cyclophosphamide + Corticosteroids	Others
Large arteries	+++	-	+
Medium arteries	+	++	++*
Small vessels and medium arteries	+	+++	-
Small vessels	+	-	++

* Includes plasmapheresis, anti-viral therapy for hepatitis B-associated vasculitis and intravenous immunoglobulin for Kawasaki disease
+++ most responsive
++ moderately responsive
+ some response
- not frequently used
Reproduced from Scott and Watts
(1994, British Journal of Rheumatology 33: 897-898)

Prof David G I Scott
Department of Rheumatology
Norfolk & Norwich University Hospital
Colney Lane
Norwich NR4 7UY

The Skin and Lupus

Introduction

The development of some sort of a rash is one of the commonest features of lupus and is often the first sign of the condition. Frequently, lupus of the skin is the only manifestation and can persist for decades. There are times when recognising the rash and typical histology can clinch the diagnosis. While only rarely life-threatening, involvement of the skin by lupus makes a major contribution to the poor health and psychological trauma frequently felt by people with the condition.

The French physician, Pierre Cazanave, published a clear description of chronic cutaneous lupus in 1833 based on the observations of his professor and mentor, Laurent Biett. Later, in 1851, Cazenave coined the term "lupus erythematosus". It is generally thought that Ferdinand von Hebra, another distinguished 19th century physician, was the first to liken the distribution of the lupus rash on the cheeks and the bridge of the nose to that of a butterfly. It was his son-in-law, Moriz Kaposi, who recognised that some patients with lupus erythematosus could become ill and develop systemic complaints. The butterfly rash is still recognised as the classic sign of lupus but actually only occurs in the minority of patients.

A wide variety of skin lesions can be seen, some of which are highly characteristic of the disease. As shown elsewhere in this guide, lupus presents a broad spectrum of disease. Thus, the spectrum of skin involvement ranges from chronic, localised cutaneous disease to lesions accompanying systemic lupus. Rather analogous to leprosy, expression of lupus reflects the response of the immune system, apparently with cell-mediated mechanisms predominating at the localised cutaneous end of the spectrum and striking serological features at the systemic end including potentially pathogenic autoantibodies which, possibly, have a direct role in certain skin lesions.

Skin manifestations

More than two thirds of those with SLE develop a rash. However, for every patient with SLE there are two or three where lupus remains confined to the skin. The wide variety of skin manifestations in lupus is illustrated in Table 1, which makes a distinction between lesions which clinically and histologically are characteristic of lupus and other forms of skin involvement that are not so specific for lupus *per se*, but may be seen in SLE.

The most characteristic histological feature of typical lupus involvement of the skin is an interface dermatitis with inflammation and damage to the basal cell layer of the epidermis, sometimes termed "liquefaction degeneration", due primarily to induction of programmed cell death of keratinocytes (apoptosis). Keratinocytes are normally very resistant to apoptosis and, apart from lupus, this is rarely seen in skin diseases other than dermatomyositis and lichen planus. Additional changes include epidermal atrophy, hyperkeratosis with follicular plugging and atrophy of the adnexal structures. As summarised in Table 1, lupus-specific skin lesions are often categorised into chronic, subacute, or acute based on their clinical features and, in particular, on their ability to produce scarring and atrophy. This is most florid in chronic discoid lesions and least so in the acute erythema of acute cutaneous lupus erythematosus.

Skin tests

Direct immunofluorescence of lesional skin characteristically shows granular deposition of immunoglobulin and complement components at the dermo-epidermal junction in both chronic and acute lesions. In addition, deposition of immunoglobulin and complement also occurs in non-involved skin, particularly from light exposed regions such as the extensor surface of the forearm, in systemic lupus but not in chronic cutaneous lupus. This is the "lupus band test" which has rather fallen out of favour as a diagnostic test for lupus since serological tests * generally provide sufficient support for the clinical diagnosis. However, the presence of granular deposits of IgG with or without complement components has a high degree of specificity for lupus.

* See chapter - Testing for Lupus

Types of skin lupus

Chronic cutaneous lupus (CCLE) is most often manifested as the discoid LE skin lesion (DLE). It is usually a well-demarcated lesion which begins as an erythematous papule or plaque and, as it progresses, develops increasing hyperkeratosis (scale) and scarring (Figure 1). Typically, it occurs in light exposed areas of the head and neck. As the lesion ages, there is dilatation of the follicular openings which become filled with keratinous debris (follicular plugging). Involvement of the scalp leads to scarring alopecia (Figure 2).

In most cases of DLE, the disease is confined to the skin and the ANA test is negative or transiently positive, usually in low titre. Approximately 5-10% of patients, however, develop systemic disease either at onset or later in the course. The risk of systemic disease is increased in certain morphological variants of DLE (Table 1), if multiple DLE lesions extend onto the trunk and extremities or if there are striking serological abnormalities with the presence of autoantibodies particularly characteristic of lupus. Lupus profundus describes indurated lesions due to inflammation of the deep dermis and subcutaneous fat, occurring mainly on the head, face and upper arms, often beneath typical lesions of DLE.

Lupus tumidus (Papular LE) is a less emphasised form of cutaneous lupus which also occurs predominantly in light exposed regions. It is characterised histologically by a dense T lymphocyte infiltrate with relatively minor epidermal changes. Sometimes it is difficult to distinguish this from Jessner's lesions. Warty or verrucous LE is another variant in which there is very prominent hyperkeratosis.

Subacute cutaneous lupus (SCLE) is a term used to describe a subset of patients with lupus with a very characteristic pattern of disease expression and serological findings, notably the presence of autoantibodies to the nuclear ribonu-cleoproteins, Ro and La. Affected patients are almost always Caucasian and cutaneous manifestations often dominate the clinical picture. Typically, the rash occurs in a light-exposed distribution and has an annular, polycyclic appearance (Figure 3) and heals with only minimal scarring or atrophy.

Acute cutaneous lupus (ACLE) lesions are associated with systemic disease and are frequently transient, episodic and reflect disease activity. The classical "butterfly" rash (Figure 4) is characterised by erythema and oedema of the malar skin. This occurs in about a third of patients with lupus.

Other causes of butterfly rash

A butterfly rash is not always due to lupus and certain common skin conditions can mimic lupus. Rashes commonly mistaken for lupus include rosacea, seborrhoeic dermatitis and, occasionally, allergic reactions of the skin due, for example, to cosmetics.

Photosensitivity

Photosensitivity is common in lupus and a prominent feature of the disease in approximately 40% of lupus patients. Often the rash worsens after sun exposure, but sometimes involvement of UV light is suggested by the distribution of the rash in typical light-exposed areas – the face, back of neck, ears, upper chest, backs of hands and fingers. SCLE is the most photosensitive form of lupus and patients often react to both UVB and UVA. In SLE, sun exposure can aggravate systemic symptoms as well as the rash. People with a light skin tend to be most affected. Sometimes, even visible light aggravates lupus. Occasionally, patients are affected by fluorescent tubes in the home or at work or even photocopiers, which predominantly radiate visible light.

Other cutaneous lesions

Table I lists a variety of cutaneous lesions which are seen in lupus but are not LE-specific. These manifestations tend to be a feature of active, systemic disease and include purpura, similar to that seen in Henoch Schönlein purpura, due to small vessel vasculitis. Livedo reticularis is a mottled red or bluish discoloration of the skin with a netlike pattern. It results from stagnation of blood in dilated superficial capillaries and venules and is associated with the presence of antiphospholipid antibodies and an increased risk of recurrent vascular thromboses and miscarriages.

Hair involvement in lupus

Generalised hair loss (alopecia) can accompany a flare of lupus. This is usually not permanent, the hair regrowing once the lupus has been controlled. Some patients with lupus complain of increased fragility of the hair, particularly at the front and at the sides. Hair loss can occur in patches if discoid lupus affects the scalp and is sufficient to damage the hair follicles. Hair loss of this type is usually permanent.

Treatment

Table 4 summarises an approach to treating lupus skin disease. The goals of management are to improve the appearance of the skin and to prevent scarring and telangiectasia. The emphasis is on symptomatic treatment and only very rarely is it necessary to resort to high-dose systemic steroids or immunosuppressive agents for skin disease per se. Treatment of the skin in lupus often needs a multidisciplinary approach. Involvement of a dermatologist with experience of treating lupus is invaluable, together with input from other health professionals such as a specialist nurse to help with non-medical aspects of management. The emphasis is on self-management. Adequate education about the condition itself and the goals of treatment are essential.

Experience has shown that the great majority of cases, even with severe skin involvement, can be managed with a combination of effective protection against UV irradiation, the judicious use of topical corticosteroids and antimalarial agents.

Sunscreens represent a cornerstone of therapy and in some patients with SCLE is all the treatment that is needed. Patients should also avoid lengthy exposure to direct sunlight and wear a hat and long sleeves to provide a barrier. Preparations with a high sun-protective factor are required (SPF 15 or higher) and need to be used regularly. The SPF value applies only to UVB and often total sun blocks containing zinc oxide or titanium dioxide, with a star rating of at least four, are needed to protect against UVA.

Table 2 lists some of the topical treatments for skin involvement. Topical corticosteroids can be very effective for patients with chronic or subacute cutaneous lupus. Potent preparations are often needed to begin with but excessive use of potent topical steroids can induce atrophy and follicular inflammation and should be avoided especially on the face. Stubborn lesions may require polythene occlusion and for small chronic lesions, especially on the extremities, flurandrenolone tape can be cut to size. Rarely, intralesional triamcinolone (10mg/ml) is necessary, particularly for lesions on the ears and nose. Injections should be directed as superficially as possible, but even so there is still a risk of atrophic scarring. When severe inflammation has settled, it is better to maintain improvement with medium or low potency preparations.

There is anecdotal evidence that a variety of other agents used topically can be effective in cases not responding satisfactorily to local corticosteroids. None as yet have been subjected formal randomised controlled studies. An example is the topical use of the macrolide immunosuppressants, tacrolimas and picrolimas.

If topical therapy fails, or the lesions are too extensive, antimalarials such as hydroxychloroquine can be very effective. Ocular toxicity with this drug has been greatly exaggerated and is very unusual if the dose does not exceed 6mg/kg body weight/day. Smoking reduces efficacy of antimalarials and in those who are still unresponsive it is worth trying combination antimalarials, for example hydroxychloroquine and mepacrine.

As summarised in Table 3, a number of medications, or combinations of these, have proved to be effective as second line agents in refractory cases. They are generally used in the context of severe acute systemic lupus but have been used for severe refractory skin disease per se. For example, thalidomide can be effective in difficult cases. However, tolerability is a problem even with small doses, as well as being highly terratogenetic. Sensory neuropathy is a particular problem and often limits long term use.

Scarring of the skin

When scarring or telangiectasia has occurred, especially on the face, cosmetic camouflage can be vitally important to the patient. The Red Cross provides a service to teach patients and can be accessed via a dermatologist. Disfiguring lesions may respond well to excision and grafting or even dermabrasion. CO_2 laser therapy is an alternative destructive technique.

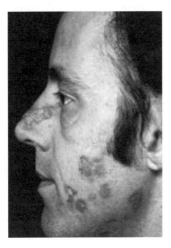

Figure 1. Discoid lupus erythematosus

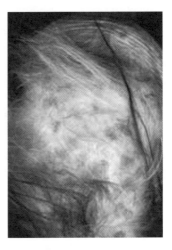

Figure 2. Scarring alopecia

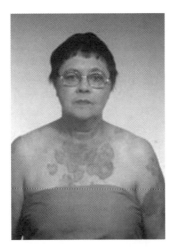

Figure 3. The typical annular rash of SCLE

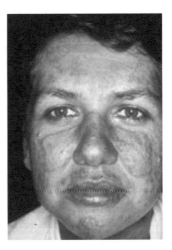

Figure 4. "Butterfly" rash

Table 1 – Skin lesions associated with lupus erythematosus

CLINICAL VARIANT	SYSTEMIC FEATURES
A. Lesions with typical LE histology	
1. Chronic cutaneous LE (CCLE)	
a) Classical discoid LE (DLE)	
i. Localised DLE	Uncommon
ii. Generalised DLE	More common
b) Hypertrophic DLE	Uncommon
c) Papular LE	Uncommon
d) Chilblain LE (perniotic lupus)	More common
e) Lupus profundus	More common
f) Mucosal DLE	Uncommon
2. Subacute cutaneous LE (SCLE)	
a) Annular SCLE	Usual
b) Papulosquamous SCLE	Usual
3. Acute cutaneous LE (ACLE)	
a) Localised ACLE ("Butterfly" rash)	Usual
b) Generalised maculopapular ACLE	Usual
B. Non-specific skin lesions	
1. Cutaneous vascular disease	
a) Vasculitis	
i. Small vessel (purpura; urticarial)	Usual
ii. PAN-like	Usual
b) Livedo reticularis	Thrombotic tendency
2. Non-scarring alopecia	Usual
3. Panniculitis	Usual
4. Bullous lesions	Usual

Table 2 – Local therapy for lupus skin disease

Corticosteroids
Tacrolimas
Picrolimas
Tretinoin
Calcipotriol

Table 3 - Drugs used for refractory lupus skin disease

Thalidomide	(CCLE; SCLE)
Dapsone	(DLE; SCLE; vasculitis; bullous LE)
Acitretin	(CCLE, especially hypertrophic LE)
Auranofin	(CCLE)
Clofazimine	(CCLE)
Pulse IV methylprednisolone	(ACLE; extensive photosensitive eruption)
High dose IV immunoglobulin	(Refractory skin disease)
Immunosuppressive agents	(Refractory skin disease)

Incl: azathioprine
          methotrexate
          ciclosporin A
          mycophenolate
          rituximab

Table 4 - A suggested algorithm for treating cutaneous lupus

Supportive	regular sun screen
	cosmetic camouflage
Mild, localised	topical corticosteroids
Severe, widespread	topical corticosteroids plus hydroxychloroquine
Refractory	hydroxychloroquine plus mepacrine

↕

dapsone or retinoids

↕

thalidomide or auranofin or clofazamine

↕

azathioprine or methotrexate or mycophenolate
plus corticosteroids

↕

IV immunoglobulin or rituximab

Prof Peter Maddison
North West Wales Rheumatology Service
Ysbyty Gwynedd
Bangor LL28 5SL

The Joints and Lupus

Introduction

Arthralgia is a frequent symptom in patients with lupus and is often the presenting symptom. Not all patients with arthralgia will progress to a true arthritis. However, arthritis is included as an item in the 1982 American College of Rheumatology (ACR) revised classification criteria for lupus and is defined as a non-erosive arthritis, involving two or more peripheral joints, which is characterised by tenderness, swelling and/or effusion.

Prevalence

The musculoskeletal system is the most commonly involved system in patients with lupus. Different cohorts report the prevalence to be between 50-95%. Joint pain is the commonest initial symptom, being the presenting problem in 50% patients. Fortunately, despite its frequency, joint disease is rarely serious and only 10% of lupus patients develop significant joint deformities. The known risk factors for patients with lupus developing a deforming arthropathy include secondary Sjögren's Syndrome, the presence of a positive anti-Ro antibody, an elevated C-reactive protein (CRP) and a positive rheumatoid factor (RF). Approximately 2-3% of patients who are classified as having lupus and have erosive disease will also meet the ACR criteria for rheumatoid arthritis (RA). It is important to screen for extra-articular manifestations associated with a connective tissue disease so that the correct diagnosis is made.

Pathogenesis

The joint deformities in lupus are usually due to tenosynovitis, particularly of the flexor tendons, rather than intra-articular synovial hypertrophy and bony erosions and loss of joint space due to cartilage destruction, as in patients with RA. In lupus patients, there is also ligament laxity combined with muscle imbalance which contributes to the development of the deformity. Musculoskeletal ultrasound and MRI scans are more sensitive at detecting joint abnormalities compared with conventional radiography. MRI findings reported in lupus patients include tenosynovitis, capsular swelling, joint effusions and, sometimes, erosions. As in patients with RA, an MRI scan is more sensitive at detecting erosions in patients with lupus compared with conventional radiography. In some studies, a high proportion of patients with established lupus had erosions on MRI scan compared with 4% on conventional X-rays.

The synovium of patients with lupus has not been studied extensively but synovial membrane hyperplasia, microvascular changes, fibrin deposition and perivascular infiltrates have been documented. Interestingly, there is little cartilage or bone destruction, which reflects the altered cytokine profile, particularly reduced levels of IL1 and IL6. The low cytokine levels within the joint mean that there is little circulating pro-inflammatory cytokine and, therefore, the liver is not stimulated to produce an elevated CRP. A common differentiation between lupus and rheumatoid arthritis is that lupus patients usually have a normal CRP and elevated ESR whereas RA patients have both an elevated CRP and ESR.

Symptoms

Patients with lupus arthritis typically suffer from stiffness, pain and swelling. These symptoms are usually worse in the morning and reflect active inflammation. It is notable that some patients may experience inflammatory-sounding joint pains for a considerable time without objective physical signs of inflammation i.e. without swelling. This may delay diagnosis and can make treatment difficult. The arthritis or arthralgia may be persistent, intermittent or flitting from joint to joint, but is typically symmetrical.
The metacarpophalangeal (MCP) and proximal interphalangeal (PIP) joints are the most commonly affected. Other joints frequently involved include the wrists, knees, elbows and shoulders.

The hand

A patient with lupus may have rheumatoid-like deformities including ulnar deviation, swan neck deformities and subluxation of the thumb, MCP and PIP joints - see figures 1-3. This pattern of deformity is characteristic of Jaccoud's arthropathy. The changes are usually reversible since they are due to tendon involvement rather than synovial damage and so the patient does not usually require or benefit from joint surgery. Importantly, X-rays of the hands of lupus patients rarely (approx 4%) show erosions – see figure 4.

The foot

The common deformities seen in the foot are hallux valgus, metatarsal phalangeal subluxation and hammer toes.

The neck

Atlanto-axial subluxation can occur as a rarity in lupus patients. It has been associated with corticosteroid use, longer disease duration, Jaccoud's arthropathy and chronic renal failure.

Extra-articular associations

There is an increased prevalence of median nerve compression producing carpal tunnel syndrome in lupus patients, as in other patients with inflammatory arthropathies. Nodules occur infrequently in lupus patients. They are typically found in the small joints of the hand but also in the more characteristic areas for RA e.g. the extensor surface of the elbow. Calcinosis also occurs in patients with lupus but is less prevalent compared with patients with systemic sclerosis or dermatomyositis. Calcinosis is often only evident on X-ray.

Table 1 - Arthritis and its associated features in Lupus and RA		
Feature	**SLE**	**RA**
Peripheral symmetrical polyarthritis	Present	Present
Erosions	Usually absent (present 4%)	Often present (up to 100%)
PV/ ESR	Increased	Increased
CRP	Usually normal	Increased
Nodules	Usually absent	Present in up to 30%
RF	Positive in minority	Positive in 70%
ANA	Positive in > 90%	Positive in 20%
dsDNA	Positive in >80%	Negative

Practical Issues

Making the diagnosis

Lupus should be considered in the differential diagnosis in a patient presenting with a persistent inflammatory symmetrical arthritis. RA can also present in a similar way. Table 1 summarises the differences. A history of extra-articular manifestations e.g. a photosensitive rash, mouth ulcers, alopecia and Raynaud's is in keeping with a diagnosis of lupus.

Monoarthritis in a lupus patient

If a lupus patient has one particular active, i.e. hot, swollen and tender, joint relative to the other joints then a septic arthritis should be considered. The joint should be aspirated urgently and the synovial fluid sent for urgent microscopy, culture and also staining for alcohol and acid fast bacilli. Staphylococcus and streptococcus are the two most common causes of septic arthritis but mycobacterium tuberculosis and nontuberculous mycobacterial infections are becoming more prevalent and should be borne in mind.

Isolated hip pain

This should raise the suspicion of avascular necrosis (also known as aseptic necrosis or ischaemic necrosis of bone). It occurs in 4-9% of lupus patients. Most cases are associated with high corticosteroid use and can occur within 3 months of starting prednisolone. It is also more common in lupus patients with Raynaud's, small vessel vasculitis, fat emboli and secondary antiphospholipid syndrome. The radiological changes are best detected on an MRI. It is treated by limiting weight-bearing, adequate pain relief e.g. NSAIDs and, for a selected group of patients, by surgery. There is controversy over the value of the core decompression for early lesions but hip arthroplasty clearly has a place for end-stage lesions. Osteonecrosis also commonly occurs in the knees, in the tibial plateau and the humeral head in lupus patients.

The swollen calf: a ruptured Baker's cyst versus a deep vein thrombosis (DVT)

Both diagnoses can occur in lupus patients. Baker's cysts are more prevalent in patients with an inflammatory arthropathy and the prevalence of DVTs is increased in lupus patients due to the increased prevalence of the secondary antiphospholipid syndrome.
See chapter – The Antiphospholipid (Hughes) Syndrome

The two conditions require different treatments and potential complications can occur if the wrong treatment is given e.g. haemorrhage into the calf, causing a compartment syndrome if a patient with a ruptured Baker's cyst is inadvertently anti-coagulated. Diagnosis is aided by performing an early ultrasound/Doppler examination. The patient with a ruptured Baker's cyst should receive an intra-articular corticosteroid injection and the patient with a DVT should be anti-coagulated.

Tendon rupture

This tends to occur in the weight bearing areas e.g. the infra-patella tendon of the knee and the Achilles tendon of the ankle. This complication is associated with trauma, long-term therapy with oral corticosteroids, intra-articular steroid injections, Jaccoud's arthropathy, long disease duration and males.

Treatment
General

The priority is to provide adequate pain relief and, therefore, maintain normal function.

Non-pharmacological

Education from the physiotherapist and occupational therapist regarding joint protection and exercise is valuable in preventing joint deformity and maintaining muscle strength. Swimming, walking and cycling should be encouraged, however, rest is important during times of marked joint inflammation. The topical application of heat or cold often provides symptomatic relief to a particularly active joint. Localised severe pain may also be helped by the application of a TENS machine (transcutaneous electrical joint stimulation) unit. Splints may occasionally be useful in correcting joint deformities. Corrective tendon surgery and joint replacement may be necessary on rare occasions in very severe cases.

Pharmacological
Simple analgesics and non-steroidal anti-inflammatory drugs

Simple analgesics e.g. paracetamol, co-dydramol and non-steroidal anti-inflammatory drugs (NSAIDs) provide symptomatic relief and are the first line of therapy. There are numerous NSAIDs and most doctors tend to become familiar with just a few. Cox 2 selective NSAIDs can be used provided there are no contra-indications e.g. hypertension, ischaemic heart disease. Renal toxicity can also occur secondary to NSAIDs and so renal function needs to be carefully monitored, particularly as these patients are prone to renal impairment per se. Choosing a NSAID with a relatively long half-life or modified release formulation has advantages for the control of chronic inflammatory pain. It reduces early morning stiffness and provides better symptomatic relief and compliance. If the optimal dose of a NSAID does not produce a significant improvement after three to four weeks, then a different NSAID should be tried. A patient presenting with new onset synovitis may experience complete relief of their symptoms after taking a NSAID, thus confirming the presence of an inflammatory arthritis.

Hydroxychloroquine is effective in treating the arthritis associated with lupus as well as the skin manifestations and, therefore, represents the cornerstone of treatment in patients with lupus.
See chapter - Drug Therapy of Lupus

Corticosteroids

Intra-articular, intra muscular and/or oral corticosteroids treat lupus arthritis effectively. If only one joint is affected then an intra-articular injection is probably the most appropriate mode of administration. Intra-muscular long-acting corticosteroids are very effective in treating a flare. If corticosteroids are required regularly then the background lupus therapy should be reviewed and a change in second-line drug considered or an additional drug added. Steroids should be used at the lowest effective dose in combination with NSAIDs, antimalarials and/or other second line drugs e.g. azathioprine, methotrexate, mycophenolate. Secondary osteoporosis is a particular risk in patients taking regular oral prednisolone and should be monitored with DEXA scans and preventative therapy with a bisphosphonate should be considered according to guidelines.

Other drugs

Azathioprine and methotrexate are both effective in lupus arthritis and are corticosteroid-sparing. Patients taking these medications require regular monitoring for drug toxicity, namely marrow suppression and liver inflammation. The British Society of Rheumatology (BSR) has published recommended blood monitoring guidelines.
See chapter - Drug Therapy of Lupus

Secondary fibromyalgia

Fibromyalgia is a syndrome of widespread pain and the presence of many tender points and is associated with a poor sleep pattern. Patients with lupus can develop secondary fibromyalgia. The control of pain can be very difficult in lupus patients, particularly if secondary fibromyalgia has developed. One approach is to develop stress management/coping strategies with an exercise regime and prescribe low dose amitriptyline to modify the pain pathway, in addition to

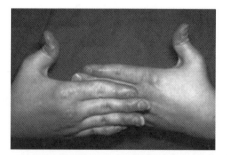

Figure 1. MCP swelling. Z thumbs and swan necking
in a lupus arthritis patient

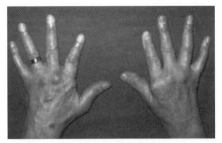

Figure 2. Subluxation of MCPs and ulnar deviation

Figure 3. Reversibility of lupus arthritis

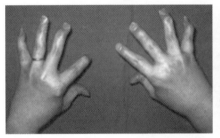 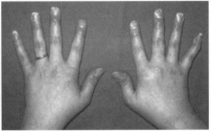

a) voluntary induction of deformities   b) returning to almost normality

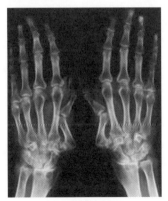

Figure 4. X-ray of hands of lupus patient showing
non-erosive arthropathy including Z thumbs

prescribing analgesics.

Dr Bridget Griffiths	Prof Paul Emery
Consultant Rheumatologist	arc Professor of Rheumatology
Freeman Hospital	Academic Section of Musculoskeletal Disease
Newcastle upon Tyne	Chapel Allerton Hospital

The Eyes and Lupus

Ocular manifestations of Systemic Lupus Erythematosus (lupus) are unusual. Broadly, they can be divided into those affecting either the front or the back of the eye or as drug effects, particularly those of hydroxychloroquine.

A. Front of the eye

(a) Keratoconjunctivitis sicca

Approximately 25% of lupus patients will have evidence of keratoconjunctivitis sicca (dry eyes). The main symptoms are of gritty, irritable, uncomfortable eyes that may be associated with some redness. Vision is unaffected; there is no pain, photophobia or discharge.

Treatment

Artificial tear substitutes, instilled as drops or a gel, usually give relief of symptoms. When selecting a treatment the main factor to consider is its viscosity. Low viscosity drops require frequent administration (sometimes more than hourly) but have minimal effect on vision. More viscous gels transiently blur the vision but are longer lasting and so may be effective when used only 4-6x/d. Highly viscous paraffin based ointments significantly blur vision and may only be suitable for night time use. A combination of a gel during the day and a paraffin at night is one popular and effective combination (Table 1).

Patients with more severe keratoconjunctivitis sicca who do not respond to these treatments will need to be referred to an ophthalmologist who will consider using preservative-free preparations, physiological tear substitutes (e.g. the hyaluronic acid based preparations), or even plugging the openings of the tear ducts.

(b) Scleritis

This is an unusual but potentially sight threatening condition and may be an important indication of the severity of the lupus. One or both eyes may be involved and patients complain of pain, often so severe that it wakes them at night. There is an area or areas of intense redness with normal visual acuity, no photophobia or discharge.

REFER URGENTLY TO AN OPHTHALMOLOGIST.

Treatment

Mild cases usually require the use of oral non-steroidals. Failure of treatment or severe cases will need systemic immunosuppression in the form of oral corticosteroids often with an immunosuppressant and, in resistant cases, pulsed intravenous methylprednisolone and cyclophosphamide.

(c) Other manifestations

Conjunctivitis and episcleritis have been described but are rare.

Treatment

Conjunctivitis can be treated with a course of antibiotic drops. Episcleritis, which may present with patches of redness, normal vision, no pain or photophobia but occasional discomfort and no discharge, may be a self-limiting condition. Oral non-steroidals, such as flurbiprofen can be effective but should only be prescribed if there are no contra-indications as a result of the lupus. Topical corticosteroids have a role in resistant cases but should normally only be prescribed under ophthalmic supervision.

B. Back of the eye

Despite the well-recognised and documented features described below, these manifestations are unusual.

(a) Retinal Disease

Retinal findings in lupus may result from several pathophysiological mechanisms, including small vessel vasculitis, large vessel occlusive disease, secondary systemic hypertension, and anaemia. Ocular complications tend to occur in acutely ill patients with active system disease.

i. Lupus retinopathy

Classic findings are cotton wool spots and retinal haemorrhages which may be found in 5 to 15% of patients. This microangiopathy probably results from the vasculitis associated with immune complex deposition in the small vessels. A prospective clinical study revealed that 88% of patients with lupus retinopathy had active systemic disease. Furthermore, lupus patients with retinopathy had a significantly decreased survival compared with lupus patients without retinopathy. Visual loss is uncommon and the patients may be asymptomatic.

Treatment

The retinopathy improves with treatment of the systemic disease.

ii. Retinal vasculitis

A few patients with lupus retinopathy develop a severe retinal vasculitis with possible progression to proliferative retinopathy. The visual prognosis is much worse with more than 50% of affected eyes seeing 6/60 or worse. The underlying process is characterised by diffuse arteriolar occlusion with extensive capillary non-perfusion and retinal neovascularisation may result. This may present as a gradual loss of vision, or sudden loss resulting from a vitreous haemorrhage secondary to the retinal neovascularisation. Tractional retinal detachment may occur. Severe retinopathy is typically associated with active systemic disease and with CNS lupus in particular.

Treatment

Immunosuppression, primarily with corticosteroids, is the mainstay of therapy.

Laser photocoagulation for proliferative retinopathy (similar to its use in diabetic retinopathy) is felt to be beneficial. Rarely, surgical intervention is required if the vitreous haemorrhage fails to clear or for retinal detachment.

iii. Large vessel occlusive disease

Branch and central retinal vein or arterial occlusions can occur. Arterial occlusions will result in a more profound, usually permanent, visual loss. Arteriolar, particularly branch, occlusions may form part of the anti-phospholipid antibody syndrome. Although venous occlusions often result in permanent loss, some may recover vision with time. Retinal ischaemia may be a complication and retinal neovascularisation may result, particularly after central retinal vein occlusion. Symptoms are of sudden, painless loss of vision.

Treatment

The patient should be monitored for any further complications, such as retinal ischaemia and neovascularization, which would require treatment. In addition, the systemic disease must be adequately controlled

iv. Hypertensive retinopathy

Typical retinal vascular changes can be seen in those patients who are hypertensive but these changes can be mistaken for lupus retinopathy and vice versa. Patients may be asymptomatic but would complain of sudden central visual loss if they developed a complication, such as a branch retinal vein occlusion.

Treatment

The changes often resolve with reduction of the blood pressure.

v. Anaemia

In some cases, peripheral, blotchy intraretinal haemorrhages may reflect anaemia combined with thrombocytopaenia, rather than the vasculitic component of the disease.

Treatment

The changes often resolve with resolution of the anaemia.

(b) Choroidal Disease

Lupus choroidopathy

Occasionally, the choroid (the layer beneath the retina) can be involved. Lupus choroidopathy results in multifocal serous detachments of the retina and underlying retinal pigment epithelium. These types of non-rhegmatogenous detachments (i.e. with no retinal hole) may be difficult to see with a direct ophthalmoscope. Visual loss is variable depending on the extent of macular involvement.

Treatment

The detachments may regress with improved control of the systemic disease.

(c) Neuro-ophthalmological Disease

Neurological complications of lupus are seen in 25 to 75% of patients. Several neuro-ophthalmological manifestations of lupus have been reported, including ischaemic optic neuropathy and retrobulbar neuritis. Ischaemic optic neuropathy presents with sudden visual loss, often associated with an inferior altitudinal field loss. This type of field loss affecting the horizontal meridian easily distinguishes it from more posterior visual pathway field defects which obey the vertical meridian. The optic disc is pale and swollen. A swollen optic disc in lupus may also be secondary to hypertension, central retinal vein occlusion and increased intracranial pressure from intracranial disease.

Retrobulbar neuritis results in a central or paracentral scotoma, red desaturation, pain on ocular movement and a relative afferent pupillary defect. The optic disc appears normal and the condition may be difficult to differentiate from that seen in association with demyelination. There is an association between neuro-ophthalmological disease and the anti-phospholipid antibody syndrome. Retrochiasmal visual problems, such as transient amaurosis, visual hallucinations and homonymous field defects have all been described.

Treatment

Systemic corticosteroids are the treatment of choice but although a return of vision would be expected with retrobulbar neuritis, it may not occur after ischaemic optic neuropathy.

ALL BACK OF THE EYE PROBLEMS SHOULD BE REFERRED TO AN OPHTHALMOLOGIST

C. Ocular Toxicity and Hydroxychloroquine

Hydroxychloroquine is frequently prescribed by rheumatologists for lupus and by dermatologists for cutaneous lupus. It binds to melanin and interacts with nucleic acids. Although irreversible retinopathy has been described, this has occurred at total doses in excess of those currently recommended. The literature and contemporary practice favour the use of low-dose hydroxychloroquine which confers minimal risk. At these levels only 20 cases of retinopathy have been reported in more than a million patients who have taken the drug; all these cases had been taking the drug for over 5 years. Combining data from case series found two cases of visually significant toxicity in over 2500 patients. Although an equivalent threshold dose is sometimes quoted for chloroquine (<3.5mg/kg/d) this is much less well established and should not be assumed to be a 'safe' dosing range. Risk increases with increasing dose, increasing duration and reduced renal function.

Hydroxychloroquine toxicity, although rare, can result in an impairment of visual acuity and central visual field disturbance. Clinically, this is seen as a granular appearance to the macula or the characteristic "bull's eye" maculopathy. At this stage the maculopathy is irreversible. Much debate exists with regards to screening for hydroxyquinolone toxicity as ocular damage is highly unusual, but when macular changes do occur they are irreversible. The 2004 Royal College of Ophthalmologists Guidelines for Screening describes recommendations for good practice in rheumatology and dermatology clinics. It recommends that the prescribing rheumatologist should ask about visual symptoms and record near visual acuity for each eye. Patients with visual impairment should then be referred to an optometrist who can refer any significant abnormality to the local ophthalmologist in the usual way. They also advise calculation of lean body weight and testing of renal and liver function to ensure safe dosing.

Table 1. Artificial tear substitutes (common types)

Group	Therapy	Examples
Low viscosity ('watery')	Hypromellose	Hypromellose Isopto Plain ® Isopto Alkaline ® Tears Naturale ® Artelac SDU ® Isopto Frin ®
	Hydroxyethylcellulose	Minims ® Artificial tears
	Polyvinyl alcohol	Hypotears ® Liquifilm tears ® Liquifilm PF ® Sno tears ®
	Sodium chloride	Minims ® Saline
Medium viscosity	Carbomers	GelTears ® Liposic ® Liquivisc ® Viscotears ® Viscotears PF ®
	Carmellose	Celluvisc ®
High viscosity ('thick')	Liquid paraffin	Lacri-Lube ® Lubri-tears ®
	Yellow soft paraffin	Simple eye ointment

Prof Philip I Murray
Professor of Ophthalmology
University of Birmingham
Birmingham and Midland Eye Centre
City Hospital NHS Trust
Dudley Road
Birmingham B18 7QU

Dr Alastair K O Denniston
Clinical Lecturer in Ophthalmology
University of Birmingham

The Mouth and Lupus

Introduction

The mouth can be affected by lupus erythematosus in a variety of ways but the most frequently occurring conditions are mucosal patches which are found in 10-25% of cases and xerostomia, which develops in up to 30% of sufferers. The mucosal lesions usually produce minimal symptoms whilst a lack of saliva causes a number of significant problems.

Mucosal patches

The mucosal lesions of lupus range from ulcerative or erythematous patches to white keratotic plaques (Figure 1). The clinical appearance is similar to both lichen planus and lichenoid reactions. The buccal mucosal is the site most frequently affected although any area of the mouth may be involved. The mucosal lesions are often painless but some patients may complain of pain. Topical steroid mouthwash, in the form of either betamethasone (0.5mg, betnesol) or prednisolone (5mg, prednesol), held in the mouth for five minutes three times daily will resolve any discomfort. The possibility that intra-oral changes represent a lichenoid reaction rather than lupus itself must always be considered since such mucosal lesions are seen relatively frequently with the use of the nonsteroidal anti-inflammatory drugs that patients with lupus may be taking. If the onset of any oral symptoms coincides with the provision of systemic drug therapy then it may be necessary to consider an alternative medication.

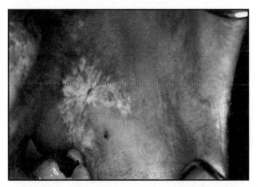

Figure 1. White keratotic patch of lupus in the left buccal mucosa.

Xerostomia (Dry mouth)

Saliva is produced by three pairs of major glands (parotid, submandibular and sublingual) and numerous minor glands scattered throughout the mouth. In health, the salivary glands produce approximately 0.75 litre of saliva in 24 hours.

Almost a third of lupus patients suffer from a significant reduction in the production of saliva which causes oral symptoms (Table 1) and signs (Table 2). In addition to being dry, the oral mucosa becomes erythematous and the tongue may appear lobulated (Figure 2).

Table 1 – Symptoms of dry mouth

Difficulty in talking
Difficulty in swallowing
Loss of taste
Altered taste
Generalised oral discomfort
Difficulty with dentures
Discomfort at the angles of the mouth

Table 2 - Signs of dry mouth

Absence of saliva or frothy saliva
Erythematous mucosa
Lobulated tongue
Dental caries, particularly at the cervical margins
Fracture and loss of dental restorations
Erythematous and pseudomembranous candidosis
Angular cheilitis

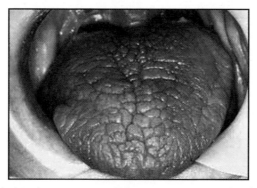

Figure 2. Lobulated appearance of the tongue as a result of xerostomia.

Investigation of xerostomia

The presence of a dry mouth can be crudely assessed by either simply looking in the patient's mouth to see if saliva is pooling behind the lower incisors or by placing the face of a dental mirror against the buccal mucosa (the mirror will stick to the mucosa if salivary levels are reduced).

In addition to these simple tests, a number of special investigations have been developed to detect reduced salivary production. Such special techniques include measurement of salivary flow rates, sialography, scintiscanning, serology and labial gland biopsy. The extent to which each of these tests is used will depend on an individual patient's history and the availability of the required facilities.

- **Salivary flow rates:** The measurement of salivary flow rates is known as sialometry. Flow rates may be assessed either as "resting" or as stimulated. Collection of saliva from the parotid glands is achieved by the use of specifically designed collection devices (Carlsson-Crittenden cups) that are placed over the right and left parotid duct orifices. The cups are held in place by suction and salivary flow collected (resting flow). For the measurement of stimulated flow rates, salivary production is encouraged by placement of 1ml of 10% citric acid on the dorsum of the tongue. A flow of at least 0.7 ml/min over a period of five minutes would be considered normal, less than this value is indicative of reduced salivary function. Assessment of flow rates from the submandibular gland is more complicated and is usually only used for research purposes.

- **Sialography:** Sialography is a method of demonstrating the structure of the salivary duct network of either the submandibular or parotid gland. The technique is based on the infusion of a water-based radio-opaque contrast medium into the main excretory duct. The medium is usually introduced using a syringe and polythene cannula inserted into the excretory duct orifice. Radiographs, consisting of a lateral oblique and antero-posterior view, are taken whilst the patient feels the gland filling. Sialography is an invaluable method of demonstrating structural abnormalities within the salivary tissues. A "snow storm effect", known as sialectasis, is a characteristic finding in lupus due to pooling of the medium within the gland. Sialography is basically a safe and simple procedure, the only contra-indications being allergy to iodine or the presence of acute infection in the gland.

- **Scintiscanning:** Radioisotopic study of salivary glands is based on the ability of active tissues to selectively uptake radioisotopes from the bloodstream. The isotope is introduced intravenously and the head/neck subsequently scanned by methods which are able to pick up isotopic emissions. This technique allows measurement of uptake and, therefore, provides an assessment of salivary gland function.

- **Serology:** Immunological investigation of venous blood can be used to demonstrate the presence of specific autoantibodies associated with salivary gland disease including anti-Ro (SSA), anti-La (SSB) and anti-salivary duct antibody.
- **Labial gland biopsy:** Sjögren's Syndrome comprises of dry mouth and/or dry eyes in combination with a connective tissue disorder, such as lupus. Histopathological examination of the minor salivary glands within the lower lip is the single most specific diagnostic test for confirmation of Sjögren's Syndrome and, therefore, can be used to confirm a diagnosis of lupus. The minor glands lie superficially behind the lower lip and can be collected simply under local anaesthesia by making a linear excision through the labial mucosa. At least five lobules of salivary tissue should be obtained since not all minor glands show the histopathological features of the condition.

Treatment of xerostomia

Treatment of dry mouth must not only involve attempts to replace the lack of saliva by the use of salivary substitutes or stimulants but should also include measures to minimise secondary problems, in particular dental caries (Figure 3).

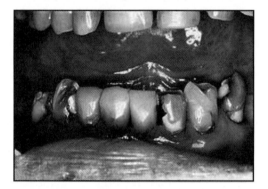

Figure 3. Fracture of dental restorations and caries due to xerostomia.

- **Salivary substitutes and oral care systems:** A number of salivary substitutes, based on either methylcellulose or gastric mucin, are available (Table 3).
- Oral care systems have also been developed and include Biotène oral balance, BioXtra, Salinum, Saliveze, Salivix and SST. Details on these formulations are provided in the British National Formulary. In addition, Biotène have a range of products that may be used in improving oral hygiene in patients with xerostomia and Oramoist produce a mouth moistening lozenge and spray.

Table 3

Substitute	Base	Comments
Artificial saliva BNF	Methylcellulose	Cheap
Glandosane	Methylcellulose	Low pH, not suitable for dentate patients
Luborant	Methylcellulose	Good pH, contains fluoride
Saliva Orthana	Mucin	Good pH, contains fluoride

Although the use of salivary substitutes may appear to offer a simple answer to the problem of dry mouth, any benefit gained is usually short-lived and, consequently, patients often resort to the use of salivary stimulants as an alternative.

- **Salivary stimulants:** A number of methods of stimulating secretion of saliva have been suggested. Many sufferers of xerostomia resort to eating traditional boiled sweets in an attempt to relieve the dryness. However, it is important to tell such patients to stop this habit since the sugar intake will dramatically encourage dental caries. Saliva flow can be safely encouraged by the use of sugar-free chewing gum or diabetic sweets. Pilocarpine is a drug that has been recommended for the treatment of dry mouth following radiotherapy and has also been used in patients with lupus. Pilocarpine can be given in tablet form at a dose of 5mg two or three times a day. However, although pilocarpine does increase salivary flow it also results in excretion by other exocrine glands and patients complain of excessive sweating or tear production. Such unwanted side effects combined with a number of medical contraindications or other side effects limit the usefulness of pilocarpine. A glycerine and lemon based mouthwash can be effective in edentulous patients although it must not be given to sufferers who have natural teeth since the low pH will encourage dental caries.
- **Oral hygiene:** Rigorous oral hygiene measures and preventive regimens, especially topical fluoride therapy, should be instituted as reduced amounts of saliva will predispose to an increased incidence of caries. In addition, it is essential that patients remove any dentures at night and clean them daily with soap using a small soft brush to dislodge food debris.
- **Fluoride mouthwash:** The use of a daily mouthwash containing sodium fluoride 0.05% will help reduce dental caries.
- **Dietary advice:** The patient should be asked to complete a diet diary over a four-day period (including a weekend). Subsequent dietary advice must concentrate on minimising cariogenic items, particularly sweetened drinks including tea and coffee.
- **Other measures:** Dry or cracked lips can be improved by use of a petroleum-based ointment such as vaseline. Patients who complain of thick

or sticky saliva may gain some relief from the regular use of a mouthwash consisting of baking soda (1 teaspoon) and salt (1/2 teaspoon) in water (1 litre). Interestingly, symptoms of dry mouth have been anecdotally reported to respond to the provision of evening primrose oil at a dose of 1000mg daily. The use of drugs that are known to reduce salivary flow, in particular tricyclic antidepressants, such as dosulepin and amytriptyline, should be avoided in patients with dry mouth.

Infection

Approximately 40% of the adult population harbour candida in their mouths as part of the commensal oral flora. Reduced salivary flow can lead to an increase in the numbers of candida resulting in opportunistic oral candidoses. The clinical presentation may be either white pseudomembranes (thrush) or erythematous atrophic areas of mucosa. Candidal infections are particularly frequent if the patient wears dentures. Topical antifungal agents are of little or no benefit in the management of oral candidosis and, therefore, it is preferable to provide a seven-day course of systemic fluconazole (50mg daily). The need for denture hygiene should be stressed if there is evidence of candidal infection. Full dentures should be placed in a dilute solution of hypochlorite at night for approximately three weeks. Partial dentures with metal components should be placed in chlorhexidine.

Opportunistic bacterial infection may develop in the salivary glands, particularly the parotid glands, due to reduced flow of saliva down the excretory duct. Acute infection presents as a painful swelling of the affected gland accompanied by a discharge of pus at the main duct orifice. Oral amoxicillin is the antibiotic therapy of choice whilst erythromycin should be used in patients with a hypersensitivity to penicillins.

Prof Michael A O Lewis
Professor of Oral Medicine
School of Clinical Dentistry
Cardiff University
Heath Park
Cardiff CF14 4XY

The Feet and Lupus

Introduction

Foot problems in lupus patients can involve any of the tissue structures within the foot (Table 1). Joint problems can lead to hallux valgus, forefoot spread and clawed or hammered toes. A high incidence of bunions and calluses has been found with these deformities along with associated pain and tenderness. Foot deformities may not be regularly reported since they are hidden and are possibly less disabling when compared to hand or finger deformities and cannot always be attributed to lupus since they are also widespread in the general population. Serious joint deformity is rare, however, over 80% of patients with Jaccoud's arthropathy of the hands have been described as having 'lupus foot' with similar abnormalities to those found in the hands, i.e. paratendonitis, synovitis, deformity and subluxation in the toes and metatarsophalangeal joints (MPJs).

It is important to note that lupus foot problems may be compounded by the dermatological complications of lupus. Neurological and circulatory problems such as Raynaud's phenomenon and vasculitis are common with possibly serious consequences such as digital gangrene. Steroid therapy further increases the risk of infection and peripheral ulceration and so any lupus patient should warrant 'high risk' podiatry care.

Table 1 - Foot problems in LUPUS

Vasculitis

Peripheral vascular disease

CNS & Peripheral neuropathy

Raynaud's phenomenon

Chilblains

Hypersensitivity

Arthritis

Jaccoud's arthropathy

Osteonecrosis

Tendonitis

Myositis

Nail dystrophy

Nailfold problems

Hyperkeratosis

The range of podiatric problems

Two thirds of lupus patients have one or more radiographic abnormalities in their feet, mainly subluxation (37%), diffuse osteopenia (29%) or cystic changes (20%). Joint involvement is usually symmetrical often presenting in the knees, ankles, MPJs or proximal interphalangeal joints (IPJs). There is usually tenderness and sometimes swelling although there is often a lack of objective signs of inflammation. Synovitis with effusions is common and deformity is often of the reducible type found with Jaccoud's athropathy although osteophytic lipping and calcification of digital joint capsules have been seen. Repeated synovitis may cause a deviation and subluxation of the MPJs, with resulting plantar pressure lesions, similar to the pattern found in rheumatoid arthritis. Foot problems tend to be worse in patients with severe hand problems and the severity increases with time.

Musculo-skeletal problems include painful tenosynovitis and tendonitis. Tendon rupture, particularly in weight bearing areas, has been reported — usually as complication of local or systemic corticosteroids. Plantar fasciitis is common and in some cases may even be a prodrome of lupus. Hypersensitivity of minor skin and nail lesions is frequently found. Peripheral neuropathies may occur from transverse myelitis and mononeuritis multiplex due to arteritis possibly causing major loss of foot function, although this is very rare. Myalgia has been seen as a result of myositis in 50% of lupus patients and gait problems can arise from muscle atrophy and weakness around the pelvis and upper leg.

Around 25% of patients have nail changes, often onycholysis or complete loss of the nails, growth may be slow and atrophic with pitting. Periungual erythema with telangiectasia can lead to skin atrophy around the nail and thickening of the nail plate with transverse and longitudinal ridges — often associated with acute phases of disease or with Raynaud's phenomenon. It has been suggested that the pattern of nail capillaries might demonstrate an evolution from undifferentiated to a specific collagen disease. The lupus patient often has tortuous, meandering capillaries with a prominent subpapillary plexus. Callus formation in the nail sulcus (onychophosis) is a common complaint but seems especially painful in lupus and can lead to infarcts and ulceration. Onychophosis can lead to an ingrown toenail as the patient tries to cut down the side of the nail, in an attempt to relieve the pain, causing a spike or wedge of nail to become embedded in the nail sulcus leading to further complications such as infected hypergranulation tissue.

Corns and callus due to mechanical stress on dysfunctional feet, with joint subluxations and toe deformities, form a large proportion of the work in routine podiatry clinics, however, the pain reported by lupus patients is often disproportionate to clinical observations and experience from non-lupus patients. Hyperkeratotic papules have been described as 'exquisitely tender' and lesions vary from inflamed weeping lesions to anhidrotic fissures. The pain can be severe and difficult to reduce with analgesics. Thrombocytopenia may cause haemorrhagic bullae and transient bullae may have caseous discharges. Purpura, discoid plaques, and erythematous macules or papules may be present and, unusually, massive hyperkeratosis with an underlying caseous layer has been described. Atrophy of the epidermis, degeneration of the dermal-epidermal junction, dermal oedema with inflammatory infiltrate and fibrinoid degeneration of the connective tissue have also been found.

Vascular complications may cause the most concern in the lower limb (Table 2), although major ischaemic problems are rare. Chilblains are common and it has been suggested that DLE patients with persistent chilblains may be at risk of developing systemic lupus. The reported incidence of Raynaud's phenomenon varies but is probably about 15-20% although it has been reported to precede lupus in a significant number of cases. This digital vasospasm may have an inflamed, cyanotic or ischaemic presentation and is frequently associated with chilblains but can lead to gangrene and amputation if not treated soon enough. The risk of digital necrosis is further increased in patients with APS due to hypercoagulation. Thrombophlebitis has been found in 10% of patients and deep vein thrombosis can also be a recurrent problem. Vasculitis, when it occurs, commonly affects small blood vessels, arterioles and post-capillary venules, forming papular, erythematous and purpuric lesions. This may also lead to splinter haemorrhages and small tender infarcts, particularly around the nail fold and in the lower leg. Slowly healing ulcers may form over areas prone to pressure or trauma such as the malleoli. Macrovascular occlusive disease has been reported in a very few cases leading to gangrene and lower limb amputation or arterial bypass.

Table 2 - Possible Lower Limb Vascular Problems

Teliangectatic lesions
Dermal Vasculitis
Thrombophlebitis
Raynaud's phenomenon
Livido Reticularis
Chronic Ulcers
Peripheral Gangrene
Dermal infarcts (similar to those in Degos Disease or Atrophe Blanch)

Treatment of the Foot in Lupus

The key aims in the treatment of the feet of any high risk patient must be prevention of serious complications, reducing pain and increasing mobility. The risk of ulceration will be increased several times if impaired circulation co-exists with foot deformities. Orthopaedic and neurological problems will lead to gait abnormalities, shoe fitting problems and increased pressure on the feet. Increased sensitivity will cause more pain whilst decreased sensitivity may reduce the patient's awareness of potential problems. Increased ground reaction forces and decreased ability to accommodate these result in more dermal stress, corns, calluses and the risk of ulceration due to decreased circulation and tissue viability. Regular assessment of the feet is essential, with advice to the patient about daily hygiene, inspection and footwear. There is no need to cause alarm if the lower limb is not affected by the disease but if risk factors become apparent podiatric referral becomes essential.

Treatment may involve aseptic reduction of corns and calluses with padding or strapping to decrease stress on the affected area or even splinting to stop motion in the toes or feet. Advice on footwear or the possible provision of insoles or surgical shoes may be needed. Biomechanical control is important and orthoses may be prescribed to stabilise the foot as a result of muscle imbalance or deformity. This may prevent or reduce compensation and wear on other joints and possible traumatic vasculitis leading to necrosis. Correct nail care is also vital and periungual problems often need skilful and sensitive treatment. Partial nail avulsion may be an option where there is co-existing nail involution or cryptosis but this may be contra-indicated by poor tissue viability leaving conservative methods of nail and hypertrophied skin reduction with nail-sulcus packing as the options of choice combined with footwear and home-care advice.

Podiatric surgery

If surgery becomes necessary, considerations should primarily involve the degree of deformity and level of pain rather than the ongoing inflammatory process. Special consideration should be given to the presence of other potentially complicating factors caused by lupus, medication etc.

Despite the relative risks, lupus patients usually respond well to carefully planned, timed and supported interventions for foot deformity. Surgery can provide great benefit and pain relief when deformity is causing a high level of morbidity in an otherwise active patient.

Podiatric Referral

The treatment of podiatric problems needs to be wide ranging and will frequently call for a multi-disciplinary approach with professionals such as wound care nurses, physiotherapists and orthotists, monitored by a specialist in connective tissue disease. More serious problems can be avoided by early examination, preventative treatment and advice. This has already been found to be cost effective and to reduce morbidity and amputation with other disease processes such as diabetes. There is some disparity between podiatry departments in those patients accepted for treatment and the service provided, however, it is common practice to see 'at risk' patients, particularly as a result of impaired circulation.

Table 3 - Risk Factors Affecting the Lupus Foot

Arthropathy and deformity

Neuropathy

Haematological disease

Vascular disease

Oedema

Cortico-steroid and other drug therapy

Stephen Miller
Podiatry Manager
Dudley PCT & Matthew Boulton College
   of Further & Higher Education Birmingham

Mrs Helen Williams
Consultant in Podiatric Surgery
The Foot Centre
West Midlands Hospital

Pregnancy, Contraception and HRT in Lupus

Introduction

Lupus is a disease that is at least ten times more common in women than in men. It most frequently presents during the reproductive years but can develop at any age from 18 months to 90 years. There has been concern that estrogen can exacerbate the disease following studies in mice and humans. In the past, there was considerable concern that lupus would flare during pregnancy with adverse effects for both the mother and baby. Until about ten years ago, women were often counselled to avoid pregnancy if they suffered from systemic lupus. It is now realised that this advice should be modified depending on the type of disease that the woman has and the type of drugs that she requires to control it. Preventing pregnancy with contraception is also an important area for consideration. Women who enter the menopause often wish to consider hormone replacement therapy. These issues will also be discussed in this chapter.

When should a woman with lupus become pregnant?

The best time for a woman with lupus to become pregnant is when her disease has been inactive for at least 6 months and she has been on stable therapy with low dose prednisolone (10mg or less/daily), hydroxychloroquine and/or azathioprine if needed. It is particularly important that renal and neurological disease are stable before a woman becomes pregnant as these conditions can have very serious consequences if they deteriorate during pregnancy. It is also important to consider other drugs that the woman may be taking and to ensure that these are also appropriate for pregnancy before the woman becomes pregnant. For example, ACE inhibitors should preferably be stopped before pregnancy or, at the latest, when pregnancy is confirmed by positive pregnancy test. Similarly, warfarin needs to be changed to oral aspirin and subcutaneous heparin when the woman becomes pregnant. However, it is not practical to maintain a woman on subcutaneous heparin for many months whilst she tries to become pregnant as well as during pregnancy. Proton pump inhibitors should be switched to ranitidine as there is much more safety data for the use of ranitidine in pregnancy.

What is the risk of lupus flare during pregnancy?

Studies have shown variable results with some showing an increased rate of lupus flare during pregnancy and others showing no increase in the rate of flare compared to the non-pregnant state. Even the studies that have shown an increase in flare rate during pregnancy have found that these are usually mild or moderate flares involving the skin and joints predominantly, rather than renal disease, providing that the woman is stable before pregnancy. Patients with inactive lupus prior to pregnancy have the least risk of developing lupus flare during pregnancy.

Renal disease can deteriorate during pregnancy, particularly if it has been active at the start of pregnancy and can be confused with pre-eclampsia with which it can also co-exist. It is very important during pregnancy to identify whether changes in clinical state are due to active lupus disease, physiological or pathological changes associated with pregnancy, or some other co-morbid condition. Patients should be regularly reviewed by their physician as well as by their obstetrician. Some pregnant patients (without lupus) develop bland effusions of the knees during pregnancy, carpal tunnel syndrome, proteinuria with hypertension and ankle swellings due to pre-eclampsia, or non-specific arthralgia and myalgia without having evidence of a lupus flare. To diagnose a lupus flare there must be an overt lupus rash (photosensitive or not), inflammatory synovitis affecting the joints with tenderness and/or swelling, hair loss or mucosal ulceration. To diagnose lupus nephritis during pregnancy there should be cells and/or casts in the urine and usually a marked increase in proteinuria before a rise in blood pressure. In pre-eclampsia blood pressure usually rises before the onset of proteinuria.

Greater confidence that lupus is the cause of a flare including increased proteinuria is obtained if there is a simultaneous rise in anti-double stranded DNA antibodies and a fall in complement C3 and C4 protein. Complement protein C3 and C4 normally rise during pregnancy so even remaining low in the normal range can be considered abnormal in the later phase of pregnancy and any fall at all of 25% or more should be considered an indicator of active disease during pregnancy. The measurement of ESR is not reliable in pregnancy as it rises non-specifically in all patients.

Treatment of lupus flare in pregnancy

Lupus patients whose disease becomes more active in pregnancy can have an increase in their prednisolone dose or start low dose prednisolone for the first time. Prednisolone is largely inactivated by an enzyme in the placenta and very little reaches the baby. However, prednisolone, particularly at doses above 10mg per day, can be associated with an increased risk of hypertension, pre-eclampsia, diabetes mellitus, infection, osteoporosis and premature delivery. Azathioprine and hydroxychloroquine do not appear to harm the baby from a number of studies, although there are very few controlled trials. Evidence suggests that the outcome for mother and baby is much better if the mother's disease is prevented from flaring by continuing these drugs or starting them if the disease flares during pregnancy, rather than by stopping the drugs which used to be the practice in the past. In contrast, drugs such as methotrexate and cyclophosphamide must be discontinued at least 3 months before pregnancy because they are teratogenic and they should not be started during pregnancy. The same applies to mycophenolate mofetil. New biological agents such as rituximab should be stopped preferably 12 months before pregnancy as there is so little data about the use of these agents in pregnancy. If the patient has been exposed to lefluonamide there are specific procedures that need to be undertaken to wash out the drug.

Other complications that can affect the mother with lupus in pregnancy

1) The most important complication of lupus disease that can affect the mother is thrombosis. All women with lupus are at increased risk of thrombosis, particularly those with anti-phospholipid antibodies (usually measured as anti-cardiolipin antibodies or lupus anticoagulant on two occasions at least 6 - 12 weeks apart). Anti-phospholipid antibody syndrome is characterised by recurrent venous or arterial thrombosis and recurrent miscarriages or other adverse obstetric history such as premature delivery, pre-eclampsia or still birth. Patients with a history of anti-phospholipid antibody syndrome are likely to require subcutaneous heparin and oral aspirin throughout pregnancy. Patients with recurrent miscarriages alone, particularly in the first trimester, may be treated with just aspirin. Some units may also use aspirin to prevent thrombosis and pre-eclampsia in patients without anti-phospholipid antibodies.

2) Lupus patients on steroids and subcutaneous heparin during pregnancy are at increased risk of osteoporotic fractures and are often treated with calcium and vitamin D_3 during pregnancy, although there is no evidence that this will reduce the risk of fractures. Fortunately, the fracture risk is small, except for women who are on very high dose steroids and/or have had many courses of subcutaneous heparin.

3) There is also an increased risk of diabetes mellitus in patients who have been given steroids, especially those on 10mg prednisolone/day or more during pregnancy. Many units will arrange a glucose tolerance test during the second trimester of pregnancy to look for evidence of impaired glucose tolerance.

Foetal outcome in lupus pregnancy

1) There is an increased risk of miscarriage and still birth in patients with lupus. The risk is greatest in those with a history of previous foetal loss due to either miscarriage or still birth, particularly in those with anti-

phospholipid antibodies or active disease during pregnancy. In the past there was some data suggesting that patients with a history of renal disease were more at risk from foetal loss, but more recent studies have not confirmed this observation, probably due to changes in treatment during pregnancy.

2) Premature delivery is more common in women with lupus. This is a delivery under 38 weeks of gestation. The delivery is sometimes spontaneous, but more often induced due to concerns about poor foetal growth. Impaired foetal growth (restricted intraruterine growth restriction) may herald the risk of miscarriage or still birth. Once the baby is mature enough to be delivered and maintained on a neonatal special care baby unit, it may be advisable to consider induction of pregnancy or even emergency caesarean section in order to deliver the baby before it dies in utero. Premature delivery is also sometimes required to protect the health of the mother in case of pre-eclampsia, particularly if it is progressing to eclampsia or if she has very severe lupus disease requiring treatment with cytotoxic agents such as cyclophosphomide. If intrauterine growth restriction is detected during the pregnancy and the mother is known to have lupus anticoagulant and/or anti-cardiolipin antibodies a case may be made to start subcutaneous heparin but intervention during pregnancy has not yet been studied to determine whether or not this will improve the outcome. All the existing studies to date are on the prevention of miscarriage and still birth by treating patients from early in pregnancy based on their medical history.

3) **Congenital abnormalities**

Major abnormalities occur no more frequently in the babies born to mothers with lupus than other women, providing that the woman is only taking approved drugs such as prednisolone, hydroxychloroquine and azathioprine for her lupus. There is a documented increase in the rate of major congenital abnormalities in patients treated with cyclophosphomide, methotrexate and probably mycophenolate mofetil, although, to date, there is very little data on this drug.

The most common congenital abnormality that can be related to lupus erythematosus is congenital heart block. This occurs in approximately 1% of lupus patients with anti-Ro or anti-La antibodies and is due to transmission of anti-Ro and/or anti-La antibodies between 16 and 28 weeks of pregnancy. Transmission of these antibodies cannot occur before 16 weeks. Transmission may occur later but the development of congenital heart block is usually detected by week 28, although it can occasionally be observed to start later than this and even after birth. Women who are known to have anti-Ro or anti-La antibodies should have foetal heart rate screening from week 16 onwards by their midwife or hospital unit. A few babies will die in utero due to congenital heart block and related cardiac complications. The majority that are born do well. However, about 30% will require a pacemaker during the first month of life, another 30% will require a pacemaker during the first year of life and a further approximately 30% will require a pacemaker by the age of 10 to 12 years.

Children have no other evidence of disease due to the transplacental passage of antibodies apart from the occasional presence of a neonatal lupus rash and, very rarely, low platelets or thrombosis. Neonatal lupus rash does sometimes occur in babies born to mothers with anti-Ro and/or anti-La antibodies after delivery when they have been exposed to sunlight or UV light (for example for the treatment of jaundice). If a mother has had a previous baby with congenital heart block, the risk of a subsequent baby having this complication is about 20%. If a mother has a baby who previously had neonatal lupus rash, the risk of neonatal lupus rash in the subsequent pregnancy is about 10% and the risk of congenital heart block is about 20%. Low platelets are rare but most common in babies born to mothers with anti-phospholipid antibodies or a history of immune-mediated thrombocytopenia.

Contraception

Although recent studies have shown no increased risk of serious flare in patients with lupus being treated with estrogen-containing contraceptives, it is still advisable to be cautious about the use of these agents in women with lupus. It should be particularly noted that they may increase the risk of thrombosis and women with a history of anti-phospholipid antibody syndrome should not be given estrogen-containing contraceptive unless they are very reliably anticoagulated with warfarin and have stable INR. They should be aware that estrogen will increase their risk of a further thrombosis. In general, women that have the lupus anticoagulant or anti-phospholipid or anti-cardiolipin antibodies should not be given oral contraceptives containing estrogen.

Women with lupus usually do well with progesterone-only contraception. Most women prefer the intra-muscular injections of Depoprovera to the oral progesterone-only pill which has to be taken very reliably within 2 hours of the same time each day and which is often associated with intra-menstrual bleeding. Barrier methods are to be encouraged particularly in young women not in a stable relationship as it will help reduce the risk of the transmission of infection. The Mirena coil is often well tolerated by women with lupus and in a stable relationship being associated with no increased risk of infection. Intra-muscular progesterone injections, such as Deproprovera, and the Mirena coil can be used in women with anti-phospholipid antibody syndrome including those on warfarin.

They should be advised that there is some risk of bleeding when the proges-terone injections are given and in the first few months after the Mirena coil is inserted, but that menstrual periods normally become lighter thereafter.

Hormone Replacement Therapy

Women with lupus are at increased risk of premature cardiovascular disease. They are also at risk of osteoporotic fractures, particularly if they have been treated with steroids. In the past, it was hoped that hormone replacement therapy would help to reduce the risk of both of these complications. Unfortunately, recent studies have shown an association between hormone replacement therapy and increased cardiovascular risk. As a result, these drugs should be used with great caution in women with systemic lupus erythematosus, since the risk of premature cardiovascular disease is at least as great as that of diabetics if not higher. Some patients will opt to have hormone replacement therapy for control of menopausal symptoms despite the risks of premature cardiovascular disease and the other known side effects of hormone replacement therapy (including malignancy and thrombosis). These women should only be given HRT after trials of other methods of symptom control and extensive discussion about the risks that they are undertaking. The situation should then be reviewed regularly as longer duration of exposure to HRT is associated with increasing risk of cardiovascular disease.

Conclusion

Women with lupus can often have successful pregnancies. It is very important that they receive pre-pregnancy counselling to ensure that they are aware of the risks of pregnancy and so that their drug therapy can be rationalised before they become pregnant. Those on anticoagulation with warfarin need detailed instructions about how to switch to subcutaneous heparin when they become pregnant. Planning pregnancy to be at a time when the woman has had inactive disease for 6 months or more, and is on an appropriate drug therapy, will be facilitated by discussions about contraception. In general, progesterone-only injections and the Mirena coil are most suitable for women who do not find barrier methods reliable enough. Sometimes both methods should be used. Once the woman goes into the menopause the use of hormone replacement therapy should be considered very cautiously, particularly in women with anti-phospholipid antibody syndrome who are more prone to thrombosis. The risk of premature cardiovascular disease is not well recognised in lupus patients but should be as it is at least as great as the risk in diabetics and, in most cases, hormone replacement therapy is not advisable.

Prof Caroline Gordon
Reader and Consultant in Rheumatology
Department of Rheumatology
Division of Immunity and Infection (East Wing)
The Medical School
University of Birmingham
Birmingham B15 2TT

Lupus: Complications and Associated Conditions

Introduction

This chapter considers the major morbidity associated with lupus from coronary artery disease, steroid induced osteoporosis and infection. It also considers some of the conditions which may overlap with or masquerade as lupus, such as Sjögren's Syndrome and fibromyalgia.

Complications

Coronary Artery Disease

In women with lupus, the risk of myocardial infarction is increased at least as much as in diabetes. Recent studies suggest that lupus may be the strongest risk factor for heart disease and stroke yet described. This greatly increased risk is probably not just related to antiphospholipid antibodies or steroid therapy. The usual risk factors appear to be important as well as the disease and its therapy. "Traditional" risk factors should be treated with as much attention as would be given to a patient with diabetes: advice on smoking, treating hypertension and optimising the lipid profile. Folic acid supplements may be useful to optimise the homocysteine levels especially in those on methotrexate or with renal impairment. Aim to keep the cholesterol below 4 mmol/l.

Osteoporosis

Steroid therapy above daily doses of 5mg or thereabouts tends to accelerate osteoporosis in the long run. This is all the more so when patients require steroids in higher doses. The days are long gone when patients were blanketed with steroids to avoid any expression of inflammation, but osteoporosis and it complications remain a major problem as the survival of lupus improves and patients grow older. The dose of prednisolone can be kept to a minimum by adding in other medications such as anti-malarials and immunosuppressives and by trying to reduce the dose whenever possible. Deflazacort may have some benefit over prednisolone if the 6:5 dose equivalence is genuine. Bisphosphonates probably reduce steroid-induced bone loss. There has always been some concern about the use of hormone replacement therapy (HRT) in patients with lupus, but the dose of estrogen turns out to be too small to cause exacerbations of the disease. It is in patients with a tendency to thrombosis through the presence of antiphospholipid antibody (lupus anticoagulant, false positive WR or antibody to cardiolipin) where there should still be concern. HRT is associated with about a threefold increase in thrombotic events in the general population and the worry is that there may also be a threefold increase in lupus where thrombotic events are so much more common. For the time being, it seems best to avoid HRT and raloxifene in patients with a history of thrombosis or with a positive test for antibodies to phospholipids.

Infection

Infection is a major problem in lupus and still a killer. Both disease and treatment impair immune defences and steroid therapy can mask symptoms of infection. Hence, it is often difficult to recognise whether illness and fever are due to active lupus or infection, or both. The white cell count is often low in lupus, so a "normal" count may suggest infection. The ESR is raised in either case, but it is useful to know that elevation of the CRP very often indicates infection. It is important to send off appropriate samples for culture and if in doubt seek help. Avoid sulphonamides as these may exacerbate lupus.

Associated Conditions
Pseudo-Lupus: *a sheep in wolf's clothing*

An important role for the doctor interested in lupus is to give an opinion on patients who just might have lupus. There is the patient with multiple sclerosis and dry eyes, the patient with acne rosacea and fatigue, the patient with migraine and little white spots showing up in the MRI scan of the brain, the patient with fibromyalgia and sore eyes and the patient prone to somatisation. Often these are worried people who are seeking the haven of a diagnosis and have read about lupus along the way. A positive test for antinuclear antibody (ANA) may muddy the waters further, and one must remember that ANA is a biological phenomenon occurring by chance or induced by medication more often than indicating lupus. If all the lupus antibody tests, including the lupus anticoagulant, are negative, a patient may be concerned about 'seronegative lupus', but this is a contentious area, best treated with a degree of sympathetic scepticism to avoid the slippery slope of unnecessary treatment. It remains to be seen whether patients benefit more from the grey area being painted black or white - no diagnosis may be preferable to a misdiagnosis.

Drug Induced Lupus

All too easy to forget, this is a chance to cure a patient. Minocycline is the chief culprit these days.
See chapter - Drug Induced Lupus

First Cousins of Lupus

We now recognise several entities which could at least sometimes be called lupus. Quite often there are particular autoantibodies specifically associated with these conditions.

Primary Sjögren's Syndrome is the most common autoimmune rheumatic disease after rheumatoid arthritis. Most patients present with symptoms of dryness in the eyes and mouth and there can be systemic illness. In some cases, the illness can be traced back to joint pains and rash in earlier years and a diagnosis of lupus may have been appropriate in the past. Indeed, we know that some patients with lupus will go on to develop Sjögren's Syndrome whether or not they give up their lupus features.

The blood tests linking these lupus patients with primary Sjögren's Syndrome include antibodies to the soluble antigens Ro and La, rheumatoid factor, high immunoglobulin G level and elevated ESR but with normal CRP. This constellation is not present in all cases, but there is usually enough to avoid a diagnosis of rheumatoid arthritis (where the IgG would be normal and the CRP elevated in active disease).

Other cousins include overlap syndromes such as **mixed connective tissue disease, anti-synthetase syndrome and anti-phospholipid syndrome.**

Fibromyalgia

Fibromyalgia or fibrositis has become a popular notion in general practice and on the internet just as some rheumatologists sound a note of caution. Fibromyalgia is defined as widespread pain (which is a condition reported by 10% of women) together with pain on palpation at certain test points (this tenderness also being associated with distress). Fibromyalgia is also characterised by sleep disturbance, waking feeling unrefreshed and day-time fatigue. It is often associated with functional bladder and bowel disturbance such as irritable bowel syndrome and with restless legs and the like, and there is much overlap with Chronic Fatigue Syndrome. Fibromyalgia is commoner in women, where the prevalence is about 2% in the general population (a fifth of all the widespread pain). Management includes acceptance, commiseration and support, advice on pacing and regular exercise, low-dose tricyclic drug such as amitriptyline at night and cognitive behavioural therapy.

The important point here is that fibromyalgia may complicate other rheumatic diseases such as rheumatoid arthritis, lupus and primary Sjögren's Syndrome in at least 20% of cases. This means that the assessment of pain, fatigue and increasing symptoms in a patient with lupus must take into account not just the question of depression but also of fibromyalgia.

So what are the concerns with fibromyalgia? Apart from the patient unlucky to have a bad back, two tennis elbows and a trochanteric bursa or the like, there is no physical problem in the musculoskeletal tissues to explain fibromyalgia, and the explanation lies in the brain. There are quite often psychosocial issues, somatisation behaviour and mood disturbance and it can be helpful for the family doctor to manage the symptoms in that light, rather than giving a pseudophysical label. The diagnosis of fibromyalgia may satisfy the patient and reduce consultation time and use of clinical resources, but this is at the expense of medicalising unhappiness, reinforcing a sense of chronic illness, risking missing other disease and transferring expenditure from the NHS to the Department of Work and Pensions. The good news is that fibromyalgia and widespread pain can have a better prognosis than used to be reported. They often improve or clear up within a few years.

Bullet points

1. Cardiac deaths are now a major concern:

   - Keep the cholesterol below 4 mmol/l
   - No smoking
   - Aspirin?
   - Folic Acid?

2. Osteoporosis in lupus:

   - Is the dose of steroids justified?
   - Consider adding a bisphosphonate and vitamin D
   - Consider HRT unless a risk of clotting

3. Drug-induced lupus:

   - Minocycline is now the commonest cause

Dr Robert Bernstein   Anson Medical Centre
Consultant Rheumatologist   23 Anson Road
Alexandra Hospital   Manchester
Mill Lane   M14 5BZ
Cheadle
Cheshire SK8 2PX

The Antiphospholipid (Hughes) Syndrome

Introduction

The Antiphospholipid Syndrome (APS) is a hypercoagulable disorder in which patients may develop vascular thrombosis and/or recurrent pregnancy loss. Its serological marker is the presence of antiphospholipid antibodies (aPL) (Table 1). Although initially described as a complication of lupus, it is now clear that the syndrome can occur without any other evidence of a connective tissue disease – the so-called primary APS.

Clinical Manifestations

Thrombosis, the main complication of APS, can affect venous and arterial vessels of all sizes; the consistent histopathological lesion is a bland thrombus without inflammation. The worldwide interest in this syndrome has led to its recognition in a wide variety of clinical states, leading to an increase in diagnosis. Indeed, it seems a fairly safe prediction that APS will overtake lupus in prevalence. A rough one-in-five rule seems to apply to the contribution of APS in various clinical conditions, i.e. one in five cases of recurrent miscarriage, one in five strokes in people under 45, one in five cases of deep vein thrombosis (DVT).

a   **Venous Thrombosis:** Thrombosis of the deep veins of the lower extremities has been reported most frequently. Occasionally, the first episode follows pregnancy or the use of estrogen-containing oral contraceptive pills. Thrombosis often recurs and may be accompanied by pulmonary embolism. Some patients with aPL also have pulmonary hypertension, perhaps caused by recurrent pulmonary emboli. More major venous thrombosis may involve the thoracic outlet veins or the inferior vena cava. Serious organ involvement includes hepatic thrombosis (APS is the second most common cause of Budd-Chiari Syndrome), adrenal thrombosis leading to Addison's disease, retinal and renal vein thromboses.

a   **Arterial Thrombosis:** Distinct from most other thrombophilic disorders, arterial thrombosis and accelerated arterial disease are striking manifestations of APS and are prognostically critical. Occlusions of the intracranial arteries have been reported most frequently, with the majority of patients presenting with strokes and transient ischemic attacks. Magnetic resonance imaging scans show changes that vary from single lesions to multiple widely-scattered infarcts. Cognitive and psychiatric features have been prominent in the presentation of some patients with APS. Large peripheral artery occlusions causing limb claudication, ischemia and gangrene have also been reported. The aorta may be involved, as well as vascular territories that include the liver, the kidney, the heart, the gut, the eye, the skin and even the skeletal system (avascular necrosis and bone fractures).

a **Pregnancy loss:** Recurrent spontaneous pregnancy loss is one of the most consistent complications of APS. Loss can occur at any stage of pregnancy, although aPL-related miscarriages are strikingly frequent during the second and third trimester. APS pregnancies which proceed into the second and third trimester are associated with a high incidence of pre-eclampsia and intrauterine growth restriction, placental abruption and premature delivery. Histological examination of the placenta from these pregnancies often shows thromboses of the uteroplacental vasculature and placental infarction. aPL are present in 15-20% of apparently healthy women who have suffered recurrent pregnancy losses.

a **Other features:** Thrombocytopenia is common in patients with APS but is usually mild (platelet count 75-100,000). Some patients with Evans' Syndrome (thrombocytopenia and haemolytic anemia) have been found to be aPL positive. Epilepsy is significantly associated with moderate to high titres of aPL in patients with lupus and has been described in patients with primary APS. It is possible that seizures in APS are the expression of ischemic events from vascular occlusions of small cerebral vessels. A similar mechanism may explain the association of APS with migraine. Valvular heart disease is a common, although often subclinical, association of the syndrome. Mitral valve thickening with associated regurgitation is the most common lesion. Livedo reticularis (a blotchy lacy pattern on the skin, most commonly seen on the knees, thighs and upper arms) is an important marker for APS. Some patients with Sneddon's Syndrome (a triad of livedo reticularis, ischemic cerebrovascular disease and hypertension) have been found to be aPL positive. Skin vessel thrombosis can occasionally lead to ulceration, often in the lower leg. The link between high blood pressure, renal artery stenosis and APS has now been well established.

Mechanisms of thrombosis

Despite the strong association between aPL and thrombosis, the mechanisms remain to be defined. The antibodies are directed against phospholipid-protein complexes and may have a direct effect on certain key membranes (e.g. platelets, endothelial cells). The antibodies may also affect the clotting mechanism itself or, more directly, key 'clotting' proteins (e.g. thrombomodulin, Protein C, Protein S). Several animal models have been established to study the syndrome and they are providing further insights into the mechanisms of thrombosis in APS.

Treatment

a **Management of thrombosis in APS:** Clinical experience suggests that patients with high titres of apL and previous major thromboses require long-term, possibly life-long, anticoagulation; in these patients international normalised ratio (INR) has to be kept around 3.0. Steroids and immunosuppressive drugs to reduce antibody titres have not provided long-term benefit. Bleeding complications may occur but the risk is not higher than that observed in other thrombotic conditions warranting oral anticoagulation. Many APS patients have benefited from self-testing their own INR. Small commercial machines are now available, which give an immediate fingerprick INR reading – invaluable for those with busy lives, travellers, or for those patients who live far from their local anticoagulation clinic.

a **Management of pregnancy in APS:** The management of pregnancy in women known to have APS is the subject of much debate and, as yet, there have been very few randomised controlled trials. Anticoagulation in one form or another is the preferred treatment rather than steroids (once widely recommended). The current choice lies between aspirin, heparin or both. Ideally, pregnant women with APS and a previous thrombosis should stop warfarin as soon as possible after a positive pregnancy test to prevent the development of warfarin-related foetal malformation. Subcutaneous, self-administered heparins are the thromboprophylaxis of choice with low molecular weight heparins being the preferred drugs. For patients who continue to have pregnancy losses despite heparin and low-dose aspirin treatment, intravenous gammaglobulin (IVIG) may be an option. IVIG is, however, extremely expensive and definitive proof of its efficacy is needed before endorsing its wider use.

Most authorities agree that one of the main reasons for the improving outcome of APS pregnancies is the closer obstetric surveillance. Viable APS pregnancies have a high incidence of obstetric and foetal complications, including intrauterine growth restriction, pre-eclampsia and premature birth, hence, close monitoring including uterine artery Doppler scans and timely delivery may improve foetal outcome in these women.

a **Management of patients with apL without prior thrombosis:** The controversy concerning whether or not prophylactic treatment is indicated for patients with apL who have no prior history of thrombosis remains unresolved as there are no available data to identify which patients with apL will thrombose. It is recommended that individuals with persistently positive apL tests take low-dose aspirin (75 mg daily) along with the removal or reduction of other risk factors for thrombosis (i.e. smoking, obesity, high blood pressure, hypercholesterolemia and estrogen-containing oral contraceptive pills). Hydroxychloroquine could be safely prescribed as it has been shown to be protective against the development of thrombosis in aPL-positive lupus patients.

Prognosis

Given correct diagnosis and treatment, the outlook of APS patients is good. For those with serious events such as pulmonary embolism or stroke, lifelong anticoagulation treatment is needed. If treatment is managed carefully no further clotting episodes should occur.

APS has had a dramatic impact on pregnancy and is now regarded as a common treatable cause of recurrent miscarriage. Low-dose aspirin and heparin have significantly improved the pregnancy success rate (85-90%) in women with aPL.

Table I - Classification Criteria for APS

Clinical
1. Vascular thrombosis: venous, arterial or small vessel
2. Pregnancy morbidity:
   • 3 or more consecutive miscarriages (< 10 weeks)
   • 1 or more foetal loss (> 10 weeks)
   • 1 or more premature births (< 34 weeks) due to severe pre-eclampsia or placental insufficiency

Laboratory
1. Anticardiolipin antibody: IgG and/or IgM (medium/high titre) on 2 or more occasions, 12 weeks or more apart.
2. Anti-ß$_2$-Glycoprotein I antibody: IgG and/or IgM (medium/high titre) on 2 or more occasions, 12 weeks or more apart.
3. Lupus anticoagulant: positive on 2 or more occasions, 12 weeks or more apart

---

APS is present when one or more clinical and one or more laboratory criteria occur in the same patient

Dr Munther A Khamashta
Senior Lecturer/Consultant Physician
Director Lupus Research Unit
St Thomas' Hospital
London SE1 7EH

Drug-Induced Lupus

Introduction

Systemic lupus erythematosus (SLE) is a genetically complex disease upon which exogenous agents, e.g. UV light, viral infection, can have significant influence in terms of exacerbating or precipitating clinical symptoms. Therapeutic drugs are one other exogenous influence and, given that most individuals receiving one of the, approximately 100, drugs associated with lupus inducing properties (LIDs; Table 1) do not develop a lupus-like illness, suggests genetic background is a critical player in this potentially serious side-effect. Those drugs that have reported associations with drug-induced lupus (DIL) do so to differing degrees, from relatively rigorous clinical and mechanistic investigations to more limited case reports. While LIDs can induce a syndrome similar to SLE, this often has less severe, or no, involvement of selected organs, e.g. kidneys, central nervous system. Some LIDs induce a condition more akin to subacute cutaneous lupus erythematosus (SCLE) consequently, unless stated otherwise, reference to DIL in this chapter means the term to encompass drug-induced SLE, SCLE and CCLE (chronic cutaneous lupus erythematosus). The use of the abbreviation 'SLE' means idiopathic SLE throughout this chapter.

Incidence and demographics of DIL

It has been estimated that, globally, the incidence of DIL caused by all drugs represents approximately 5 to 10% of the total number of patients with SLE. There are differences between DIL and SLE, DIL patients are generally older (50-70 years, a reflection of the increased use of some therapeutic drugs in older populations) than patients with SLE (average age at diagnosis, 29), the gender bias for SLE (9:1 in favour of females in the reproductive years) is not seen in DIL. White Caucasians may be affected by DIL up to six times more frequently than blacks, where the incidence of SLE is greater. The risk of developing DIL is much greater for doses of drug greater than 200mg/day and individuals often need to be taking these doses for several months to years before symptoms develop. The development of symptoms can be abrupt, initially presenting in a mild or limited manner but gradually worsening the longer the patient is maintained on the drug.

Clinical features of DIL

Accurate diagnosis of DIL is difficult. Ideally, to be considered a LID, a patient receiving a therapeutic compound should satisfy 4 out of 11 diagnostic criteria for SLE and the symptoms should disappear on withdrawal of the drug. However, the range of symptoms that are positive and could be usefully employed as diagnostic criteria for DIL are limited (arthralgia/myalgia/arthritis, serositis, antinuclear antibodies and anti-histone/anti-single stranded DNA antibodies). While the specific criteria used to diagnose DIL have not been formalised, there are several points a clinician should look out for if DIL is suspected in a patient:

- One or more clinical symptoms of SLE are present.
- Presence of antinuclear antibodies, particularly anti-histone antibodies in the absence of other anti-nuclear specificities such as anti-dsDNA.
- The patient had no history of SLE prior to taking the suspect drug.
- The suspect drug was taken continuously anytime from 1 month to 2 years prior to the onset of symptoms.
- Symptoms improve within days to weeks when the drug is discontinued, with antinuclear antibodies and other serologic markers slowly returning to more normal levels.

Arthralgia is the most common, often the only, clinical symptom in 90% of patients with DIL, with myalgia also common and present in 50% of patients. Fever, pleurisy and pericarditis are other characteristic symptoms, with cardiac tamponade associated with selected LIDs. Certain cutaneous symptoms are more evident in DIL compared to SLE (purpura, erythema nodosum, erythematous papules) although, generally, skin involvement is not as common and the cutaneous manifestations more frequently observed in SLE (malar rash, alopecia, discoid lesions and photosensitivity) are largely infrequent in DIL. Mucosal ulcers, lymphadenopathy, Raynaud's phenomenon, anaemia, leukopenia and thrombocytopenia are generally rarer in DIL. It is important to note, however, that the relative frequency of various symptoms can depend on the identity of the LID. As mentioned earlier, neuropsychiatric symptoms and glomerulonephritis are very rare in DIL. Although there are marked differences in clinical symptoms between DIL and SLE, the differences between drug-induced SCLE and idiopathic SCLE tend to be less marked, for example, the serological profiles between the two diseases are generally similar and DIL is also more common than SCLE.

Serology
Although there are similarities with SLE, serological changes are not identical to DIL and in many cases there can be significant elements of drug-specificity in the serological changes. These and other findings are noted in Table 2.

Drug-induced lupus: mechanistic considerations
An understanding of how LIDs induce lupus is still not completely clear, although notable advances have been made during the past few years. It seems that no single pathogenic mechanism can explain how all LIDs induce DIL, but of the possible mechanisms there are some notable features, which interestingly seem to tie in with aspects of what is known about the pathology of SLE. While some

LIDs may have lupus-inducing properties without metabolic transformation, e.g. anti-TNFα therapies, others, such as procainamide, may exert their lupus inducing effects following oxidative metabolism. A point worth re-iterating is that since most individuals do not react to the intake of potential LIDs by developing DIL, individual genetic constitution is key to determining adverse outcome, although the identities of the genetic pre-disposing factors are still largely unknown. Also, besides being of 'scientific interest', understanding the mechanism of action of LIDs is considered useful to aid understanding SLE, perhaps with a view to designing novel therapies.

Apoptosis

A central player in the pathogenesis of SLE, and probably DIL, would appear to be apoptosis, where dysfunctional cells, or those past their biological usefulness, are removed by an ordered destruction process and the contents of the cell are engulfed by phagocytosis. Apoptosis has an important role in immune function such as the deletion of autoreactive T- and B-cells and the removal of intracellular contents via phagocytosis to prevent the exposure of, otherwise immunologically concealed, intracellular contents, e.g. nucleosomal material, to the immune system. Evidence strongly suggests that apoptotic cells are a significant source of the autoantigens found in SLE. Interference with apoptosis could have profound implications for the development of DIL, through a failure to remove autoreactive T- and B-cells and/or inducing apoptosis, which, on the correct genetic background, where relatively minor perturbations in the load of apoptotic material may lead to the exposure of the immune system to ordinarily sequestered intracellular components, as these cannot be cleared effectively. This latter point is also important if the immune system is dysfunctional and is already pre-disposed to react to self-antigens. In SLE several factors that may conspire to increase apoptotic load, including defects in complement and the ability of macrophages to clear apoptotic cells and debris, along with defects in the enzyme DNAse I and serum amyloid P component, which can degrade/mask autoantigens. Several DIL may interfere with apoptosis:

Quinidine and procainamide: At therapeutic concentrations, inhibit macrophage scavenging of apoptotic debris.

Chlorpromazine: Induces apoptosis in activated lymphocytes.

Captopril and lisinopril: These angiotensin II converting enzyme (ACE) inhibitors are widely prescribed for the control of hypertension, yet the apparent expression of ACE on the surface of selected immune cell populations such as T-lymphocytes and monocytes suggests it may have functions in the biological activity of these cells. The effect of captopril may be to block activation-induced apoptosis, perhaps inhibiting clonal deletion and acquisition of self-tolerance.

Statins: These widely prescribed drugs (estimated at least ~25 million people currently) used to control hypercholesterolemia may exacerbate or trigger apoptosis. Also statins may directly modify T-cell function, possibly via inhibition of cholesterol synthesis in these cells leading to plasma membrane perturbations. Statins can promote a shift from Th1 to Th2 immune response, promoting a bias in the latter which is associated with B-cell activation/reactivity.

Anti-TNFα therapies: These agents such as infliximab, etanercept and adalimumab employ various strategies to inhibit TNFα. Infliximab, for example, has been shown to induce apoptosis in activated T-cells, induce increases in circulating nucleosomes and, therefore, may contribute to the burden of apoptotic material in susceptible individuals. Anti-TNF alpha therapy may down regulate control mechanisms for limiting B-cell hyperactivity (a feature of SLE) as TNFα is also an immunoregulatory molecule, which may be involved in the deletion of autoreactive T-cells, so the presence of elevated levels of TNFα may be beneficial in some circumstances. Serum TNFα levels can be elevated in SLE and mouse models with mild SLE may develop a much more severe disease when TNFα deficiency is induced.

Modulation of the immune system using other 'biological therapies' such as IL-2 and Type I interferons (IFN-α, IFN-ß) can have impacts for DIL -

IL-2 is a pro-inflammatory lymphokine that has been used therapeutically, but elevated IL-2 has been noted in association with a number of autoimmune phenomena and its hypersecretion has been associated with active disease in SLE.

IFN-α and IFN-ß have been associated with the clinical and serological manifestations of SLE thus, on the correct genetic background, use of these compounds therapeutically may lead to DIL in some individuals.

Epigenetic alterations

The control of gene expression in all cells is exercised at several levels, one process involves epigenetic phenomena (such process can lead to changes in gene expression that do not involve changing the inherent DNA sequence). The methylation of selected cytosines in a promoter region or within a gene can affect the expression of that gene and is an epigenetic process. The consequences of inappropriately modifying DNA methylation depends on the cell in question and where the methylation changes have occurred. The lupus-inducing actions of two well established LIDs, **procainamide** and **hydralazine**, either as their parent compounds or oxidised metabolites, may be partly explained by an interference with DNA methylation. In experimental animals, interference with T-cell methylation patterns using agents such as 5-aza-cytidine can induce a lupus-like disease, suggesting the correct maintenance of DNA methylation patterns is important to avoid autoimmunity. Both procainamide and hydralazine can similarly interfere with T-cell methylation patterns and, in so doing, alter gene expression and impact on T-cell function leading to autoimmune responses, the exact mechanism by which procainamide and hydralazine inhibit DNA methylation is slightly different for each compound but the outcome is similar, the promotion of autoimmunity. Again, comparisons can be drawn between DIL and SLE in this context, hypomethylation of lymphocyte DNA is a biochemical abnormality detected in SLE, as are defects in the same cell signalling pathway in lymphocytes affected by hydralazine. Impaired T-cell methylation leads to overexpression of selected cell surface molecules leading to T-cell hyperresponsiveness, thus signals that do not normally trigger T-cell activation do so, this enhanced T-cell function helps drive autoantibody production by B-cells.

Subversion of T- and B-cell tolerance

A critical feature of a normally functioning immune system is that it does not recognise the body's own cells or their components as foreign. In the case of the contents of the cell, these are usually hidden from the immune system, even when the cell dies, as they are removed by apoptosis. However, during B- and T-cell development, autoreactive cells do arise and these need to be kept in check so they do not enter the periphery and participate in autoimmune reactions. Mechanisms to control this include deletion of autoreactive cells by apoptosis, anergy (where the cells are not deleted but are rendered non-responsive) and an additional mechanism in B-cells, antigen receptor editing, whereby those cells that are initially reactive to self-antigens are rendered un-reactive via modification of cell surface receptors. Again, primarily studied experimentally with **procainamide** and **hydralazine**, these agents may subvert tolerance to self-antigens in both T-cells and B-cells acting either as the parent compound or as a metabolite (see next section). Intra-thymic injection of procainamide hydroxylamine, an oxidised metabolite of procainamide, in experimental animals induces an autoimmune syndrome with remarkable similarities to DIL, including elements of the serological profile of DIL. Procainamide hydroxylamine appears to interfere with the establishment of self-tolerance by preventing the induction of anergy. Ideas that the thymus may largely be non-functional in adults would not seem to be completely accurate thus this mechanism may have relevance. In B-cells, hydralazine has a negative impact on antigen receptor editing, perhaps by targeting the same cell signalling system that leads to disruption of DNA methylation by this LID.

Metabolic activation of LIDs, haptenisation and oxidative processes

All compounds foreign to the body undergo xenobiotic metabolism to reduce exposure, accumulation and facilitate excretion. Therapeutic drugs are perceived as foreign and, therefore, also subject to xenobiotic metabolism. Some LIDs may need to be metabolised to induce DIL and how an individual handles metabolism can be an important determinant, for example, selected LIDs may be shunted down a particular metabolic route, if a route that leads to generation of a non-toxic metabolite is slow or impaired. An example may be in the case of slow acetylators, where LIDs may end up accumulating and being oxidised rather than being acetylated. The oxidation products of certain LIDs may be the ultimate species that interferes with immune cell function. Activated neutrophils, via the action of myeloperoxidase, may be one such route for oxidative metabolism of LIDs, and multiple examples of LIDs have been shown to be oxidised by neutrophils to generate cytotoxic metabolites (e.g. **hydralazine, procainamide, propylthiouracil, isoniazid, quinidine, clozapine, chlorpromazine**). Once generated, these metabolites may subsequently have several effects: induce apoptosis; bind to cell surfaces making such cells targets for immune-mediated destruction; react with and modify endogenous macromolecules (haptenisation) which are recognised as foreign and processed by the immune system; modify cell surface proteins on immune cells and modify their biological function.

Oxidative stress, that is an imbalance of cellular oxidants and anti-oxidants in favour of the former, may have some role to play in SLE and DIL. Induction of excessive production of reactive oxygen species in target cells could be one way LID metabolites induce cell death. Additionally, DNA that has been modified by oxidants is more antigenic for the anti-dsDNA antibodies found in SLE and antioxidants, such as vitamin E, may positively modulate lupus-like disease in some animal models. Recent work in a mouse model has shown that deletion of a particular gene which controls the expression of a battery of genes involved in xenobiotic metabolism, detoxification reactions and protection against oxidative stress intriguingly leads to the development (predominantly in female mice) of a pathologic syndrome bearing striking similarities to SLE, with many of the clinical and serological findings. Notably, oxidative modification of biomolecules and markers of DNA and lipid oxidation are elevated in these animals and precede the development of lupus-like pathology. This may suggest that the gene itself or one or more of the genes under its control may be worthy of exploration in terms of individual susceptibility to DIL.

Table 1 (opposite)
- Differentiation between induction of cutaneous LE and SLE is not made in this table.
+ - Weak association in this instance means there are currently insufficient reports of cases to enable a firm decision to be reached, this may be because the lupus-inducing properties of some of these drugs has only recently been appreciated.

Table 1 – Identities of lupus-inducing drugs#

Proven Association		
Chlorpromazine. Hydralazine. Isoniazid. a-Methyldopa. Minocycline. Procainamide. Quinidine.		
Possible Association		
Acebutolol	Oxprenolol	
Adalimumab	D-Pencillamine	
Atenolol	Pheneizine	
Carbamazepine	Phenytoin	
Cimetidine	Pindolol	
Dapsone	Primidone	
Diphenylhydantoin	Practolol	
Etanercept	Propanolol	
Ethosuximide	Propylthiouracil	
Hydrazine	Quinidine	
Infliximab	Sulphasalazine	
Labetalol	Sulphonamides	
Lamotrigine	Thiamazole	
Levodopa	Timolol	
Methimazole	Trimethadione	
Mephenytoin	Tryptophan	
Metoprolol	Valproate	
Nitrofurantoin	Zonisamide	
Weak Association+		
Acetyl-L-carnitine	Estrogens/oral contraceptives	Nafcillin
Allopurinol	Ethylphenacimide	Nifedipine
Amidarone	Fluvastatin	Nitrendipine
5-aminosalicylic acid	5-Fluorouracil	Paclitaxel
Atorvastatin	Gembibrosil	Penicillin
Bupropion	Gold salts	Phenylbutazone
L-Canavarine	Griseofulvin	Reserpine
Captopril	Hydroxyurea	Rifampicin
Cefuroxime	Interferon-a	Simvastatin
Celiprolol	Interferon-ß	Streptomycin
Chlorprothixine	Interleukin 2	Tegafur-uracil
Chlorthaidone	Lamotrigine	Terbinafine
Ciprofloxacin	Lansoprazole	Tetracycline
Clobazam	Leflunomide	Ticlopidine
Clonidine	Lisinopril	Tocainide
Clozapine	Lithium	Zafirlukast
Debrisoquine	Lovastatin	Ziprasidone
Docetaxel (taxotere)	Methimazole	
Enalapril	Methysergide	

Table 2+: Serological and other findings in DIL and SLE

Feature	DIL* (%)	SLE (%)
Anti-nuclear Ab#	>95	>95
LE cells	>50	70
Anti-histone Ab	>95	50
Anti-[(H2A-H2B)-DNA] Ab	40-95	70
Anti-native DNA Ab	<5	30-70
Anti-denatured DNA Ab	50-90	80
Anti-cardiolipin Ab	5-20	35
Rheumatoid factor Ab	20-30	25-30
Elevated ESR	>50	>50
Elevate gammaglobulins	10-50	30
Hypocomplementaemia	<5	50

+Adapted from R.L. Rubin. Toxicology (2005) 209: 135-147.
*Based on two well established LIDs, hydralazine and procainamide.
#Ab = antibodies.

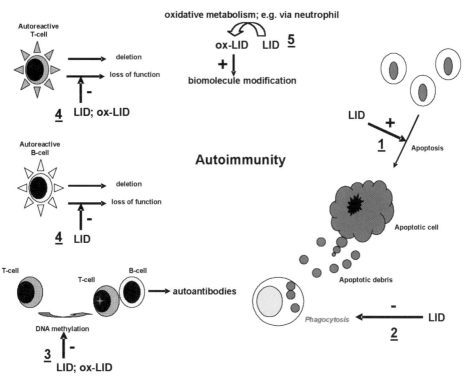

Figure 1: General overview of potential pathogenic mechanisms in DIL.

LID = lupus-inducing drug; ox-LID = oxidised LID; + = promotion; - = inhibition.
1. Induction of apoptosis.
2. Interference with disposal of apoptotic debris.
3. Alteration of DNA methylation in T-cells.
4. Interference with establishing tolerance to self-antigens.
5. Metabolism of LID by oxidative metabolism to yield biologically active LID metabolites.

Dr Mark D Evans
Non-clinical lecturer
Dept Cancer Studies & Molecular Medicine
University of Leicester
RKCSB Leicester Royal Infirmary
University Hospitals of Leicester
   NHS Trust
Leicester LE2 7LX

Dr Ash Samanta
Consultant Rheumatologist
Dept Rheumatology
Leicester Royal Infirmary
University Hospitals of Leicester
   NHS Trust
Leicester LE2 5WW

Juvenile-onset Lupus

Introduction

Although rare, juvenile-onset lupus (JSLE) causes significant morbidity and even mortality in children. It is a complex illness. It can present with such a variety of symptoms and signs that it can mimic many common paediatric conditions. This means diagnosis is often difficult to make and there are frequently significant delays in attaining specialist care. Much is inferred about the disease from adult-onset lupus. However, children are not mini-adults - their normal growth, development and evolving immune system affect the disease presentation and complicate its diagnosis and management.

What is so special about JSLE?

- **Severity of the disease** - JSLE has a more severe disease presentation than lupus in adults, with a higher incidence of major organ involvement and a more aggressive course. Paediatric patients are more likely to die in the acute phase of the illness compared to adults who more commonly die of disease complications. However, JSLE patients will also have longer disease duration than their adult counterparts and so have a higher chance of developing complications.
- **Additional management challenges** - Longer exposure time and re-exposure to carcinogenic or gonadal-toxic agents are of particular importance to patients with JSLE. Handling and bioavailability of potent immune-modulating drugs differs between adults and children. Side effects of drugs used in the management of JSLE can be particularly problematic in adolescents with JSLE. JSLE can have a dramatic impact on a child's education, social development and, indeed, their whole family.

How common is JSLE?

- There are no robust incident data for JSLE in the UK. Data from different ethnic populations from around the world put the incidence between 0.5 and 6 per 100,000.
- Approximately 15-20% of patients with lupus will present in childhood or adolescence.
- The female predominance of lupus found in adults is less apparent in JSLE. While the overall female to male ratio in JSLE is approximately 4.5:1, this difference is even less marked pre-pubertally.
- Children of any age can develop JSLE, although it is extremely rare before the age of 5 years.

Challenges of diagnosing JSLE

- Clinical manifestations of JSLE are extremely variable, from a relatively mild disease characterised by facial rash, joint pains and fatigue to a severe life threatening illness.
- These non-specific features, that could underlie a myriad of paediatric conditions, can make it a major diagnostic conundrum. Knowledge and experience of the spectrum of paediatric and adolescent disease is important as well as recognition of when features merit further investigation.
- Some symptoms of JSLE may present a long time before other symptoms. Patients may have already been diagnosed with another condition such as chronic fatigue, juvenile idiopathic arthritis, and idiopathic thrombocytopenia. Only careful monitoring and re-evaluation will enable the diagnosis of JSLE to be made.
- Although the diagnostic criteria used in JSLE are the same as those used in adult-onset lupus, they must be used with caution in JSLE to avoid over- or under-diagnosis.

What features could indicate JSLE?

- **Constitutional** – Tiredness, fatigue, lethargy and malaise are very common in JSLE. An associated anaemia may be contributory. Fever and anorexia are typically present while poor weight gain and delayed growth suggest long standing illness.
- **Cutaneous manifestations** – The characteristic facial butterfly rash is present in only about half of patients with JSLE and even then may not be diagnostic. It is often faint and typically spares the naso-labial folds. Sun exposure can, but does not always, precipitate systemic and cutaneous features of JSLE. Unlike adult-onset disease, discoid lupus is very unusual in JSLE. Raynaud's phenomenon, nailfold capillary abnormalities and livedo reticularis are all common and may precede other manifestations of lupus. While raising the clinician's suspicion of JSLE they are not diagnostic. A patient with JSLE often complains of hair thinning when brushing or clumps of hair on their pillow in the morning.
- **Musculoskeletal** – Arthritis and arthralgia occur in approximately two-thirds of patients at presentation. Symptoms, often symmetrical involving the small joints of the hands, can be transient and fluctuating with minimal objective signs on examination. Any joint may be affected. Myalgia and myositis do occur, typically in the acute sick patient, and raise the possibility of a mixed connective tissue disorder

Major organ involvement

This must be actively sought and excluded. Renal, neuropsychiatric and haematological involvement occurs more frequently in JSLE.

- Neuropsychiatric lupus, a cause of debilitating long term morbidity in JSLE, can be very difficult to diagnose and can manifest in a vast range of presentations including headache, depression, severe anxiety, aseptic meningitis, seizures, psychosis, visual disturbance or visual loss.
- Nephritis is much more common at diagnosis in JSLE than in adults. Proteinuria in an early morning urine or mild hypertension may be the only initial manifestations of significant renal involvement. However, patients may also present with severe hypertension, nephritic syndrome or acute renal failure.
- As with adult-onset lupus, JSLE can affect any organ system in many different ways. Cardiopulmonary manifestations are increasingly recognised in JSLE.

Making a diagnosis of JSLE
- The diagnosis is made from a constellation of clinical and laboratory features.
- A low index of suspicion must be maintained, particularly in a patient with varying signs and symptoms affecting several organ systems, who is not responding to usual therapies, is clinically deteriorating or in whom constitutional symptoms are prevalent.

What investigations should be carried out if JSLE is suspected?

In any child who is acutely ill in whom JSLE is suspected, an emergency referral to hospital should be made to a paediatric rheumatologist or experienced paediatrician for multi-system investigation and assessment.

In a child less acutely ill, a number of investigations may be very helpful in accumulating diagnostic evidence but should not delay referral if clinically indicated. They can also be useful in monitoring disease activity. All of these tests and more would be carried out during comprehensive assessment.

- Haematology – Anaemia is common and a Coomb's positive haemolytic anaemia and thrombocytopenia are twice as common in JSLE. Lymphocytopenia is very common and can help in monitoring disease activity.
- Acute phase proteins - Disparity in these can help in assessing disease activity reflected in a high ESR and low CRP. Elevated CRP should raise concern of inter-current infection. Both these bio-markers may be raised for other reasons which should also be considered.
- Autoantibodies – Antinuclear antibodies (ANA), the hallmark of adult lupus, are also present in JSLE but are non-specific. They must be interpreted in the context of clinical features. It is very rare that ANAs are negative in JSLE although they may be so early on in the disease presentation. There are a wide spectrum of encapsulated nuclear antibodies (ENAs) that may be present in JSLE including anti-double stranded DNA (dsDNA) and anti-Sm

antibodies. The titre of anti-dsDNA antibodies is helpful in monitoring disease activity.
- Complement – C4 and particularly C3 levels are often low in active JSLE and, therefore, routinely measured.
- Renal function and urinalysis – Blood pressure measurement and urinalysis are important in the assessment of all children with suspected JSLE. Proteinuria, haematuria or cellular casts should be followed up with an early morning urine albumin-creatinine ratio. Normal renal function does not preclude active lupus nephritis.

Interpretation of investigations and differential diagnoses
- As with adult-onset disease, there is no one diagnostic test for JSLE. All routine tests to aid the diagnosis (and long term monitoring of disease activity) are non-specific. They must be interpreted in the context of the clinical features and other bio-markers.
- The differential diagnosis of JSLE is extensive and includes infection, malignant disease, other auto-inflammatory conditions and any specific organ-associated disease. The ability to diagnose JSLE correctly, particularly in the adolescent, may be very challenging and require great clinical acumen.

Appropriate speed and referral pathway
- All children who are systemically unwell, have signs of major organ involvement, are clinically deteriorating or are not responding to existing therapy should be referred as an emergency for further investigation and assessment.
- Any child suspected of having JSLE should be discussed with or referred to a paediatrician or paediatric rheumatologist as soon as possible.

Access of specialist services – ARMA Guidelines
- Early diagnosis and access to specialist services can significantly improve outcome and reduce the risk of life-threatening events. Patients, unfortunately, frequently attend numerous appointments and specialists before a diagnosis is finally made.
- Recently published ARMA guidelines stipulate that GPs should have access to specialist units where assessment can be made by a multi-disciplinary team led by a paediatric rheumatologist. Each local District General Hospital should have a nominated paediatrician with knowledge of JSLE, access to and regular communication with regional specialist centres to whom they can refer on where appropriate. Emergency services should, therefore, be available for specialised connective tissue disease advice.

Management of patients with JSLE

There is significant paucity of evidence for therapeutic intervention specific to JSLE. Much is inferred from case series or adult studies where the disease characteristics vary. There is now an impetus from national and international collaborations to perform randomised controlled trials in JSLE.

- **Immuno-suppressive therapies** - Medications currently used to treat JSLE include: hydroxychloroquine; azathioprine or methotrexate for mild/moderate disease; mycophenolate mofetil or intravenous cyclophosphamide for severe disease or major organ involvement and, more recently, biologic therapies such as rituximab. Regular blood monitoring is important.

- **Treatment of intercurrent infection** - Patients with JSLE have an abnormal immune response as part of their disease process and all of the therapeutic agents used are associated with immuno-suppression. Any sign of infection must be actively investigated and aggressively treated.

- **Sunblock** - The highest factor sunblock is important, even on cloudy days.

- **Multi-disciplinary care** - Patients with JSLE should receive multidisciplinary care from professionals trained to address the diverse and complex issues of a chronic paediatric multi-system disease. This input is vital to address their considerable needs and concerns.

Integration of patient care in JSLE

Integration of care across primary, secondary and tertiary services is vital to improving outcome and to support children and adolescents with JSLE and their families. Patients with JSLE will require long term follow up. Travelling distances to tertiary services may be long and very disruptive to the child's education and for the family. Patients with mild disease or who are well controlled should have the opportunity to have shared care locally.

UK-wide network of care for JSLE

There are few long term outcome data on patients diagnosed with JSLE. The UK JSLE Study Group is a multi-centre, multi-disciplinary collaborative network comprising representatives from nearly all the major paediatric centres in the UK providing specialist care of patients with JSLE. It has established a UK-wide cohort of patients with JSLE to improve the knowledge base of the disease. It has set standards for the assessment, diagnosis and on-going monitoring of patients with JSLE. In partnership with LUPUS UK it is developing patient and parental information specific to JSLE and is actively pursuing a clinical trials agenda in JSLE.

Dr Michael W Beresford, Senior Lecturer (Clinical) in Paediatric Medicine
Institute of Child Health, University of Liverpool
Royal Liverpool Children's Hospital, Eaton Road, Liverpool L12 2AP

Drug Therapy of Lupus

Introduction

It would be wrong to sugest that the management of lupus is easy. The disease has numerous manifestations and each person has their own pattern of disease which can change over time, sometimes rapidly. In general, patients who present with severe lupus e.g. of the kidneys or central nervous system (CNS), and those with multiple autoantibodies tend to have persistent serious disease. Patients who present with mild disease may continue to have mild disease but, as time goes by, many will develop more serious manifestations, so it is important to consider whether any new symptom might represent a new manifestation of the disease.

Treatment of specific disease manifestations is dealt with in the relevant chapters of this book so an overview of the drug management is given here. Treatment depends upon clinical assessment of the extent of organ involvement and also of its severity (Table 1).

Assessment of disease activity

Investigations are dealt with in detail elsewhere, however, clinical assessment of disease activity is as important as the results of laboratory tests. Tiredness, fever or mood disturbance can indicate a flare of disease, as well as more obvious manifestations such as rash or arthritis. Where there is significant internal organ involvement then appropriate tests can be used to monitor disease activity e.g. serum creatinine, eGFR, urinary protein or lung function tests. Otherwise, it is often possible to identify a test which reflects disease activity in an individual patient. This may be the DNA binding level, the serum C4 or C3 concentration, the white cell count, haemoglobin or, perhaps, even the ESR. Such combined clinical and laboratory assessment helps one to decide whether it is necessary to use more aggressive treatment or, alternatively, whether the dose of medication can be reduced.

Various disease assessment indices have been developed e.g. BILAG, SLEDAI, SLAM & ECLAM and are used in specialist units. They variably assess disease activity and tissue damage and it can be difficult to distinguish the effects of currently active inflammation from those of established damage. Quality of life may also be assessed by measures such as the SF-36 questionnaire.

It is reasonable to divide lupus into mild, intermediate or severe disease, although even in mild disease symptoms such as malaise or arthralgia can be very disabling.

The main therapeutic agents are shown in Table 2, although other drugs may be used in specific circumstances and are discussed in the relevant chapters. The management of clotting problems associated with anti-phospholipid antibodies and of lupus in pregnancy are fully discussed elsewhere in this book.

Mild disease

Common manifestations are arthralgia, rashes, photosensitivity, mouth ulcers, Raynaud's phenomenon, hair loss and fatigue. Often symptoms can be reasonably controlled by analgesics and measures to reduce sun exposure, including the use of high factor sunscreens. Hydroxychloroquine is often useful in this type of disease. Mepacrine can be a useful alternative to hydroxychloroquine or used in combination with it when the response is inadequate.

Fatigue may be disabling despite control of other symptoms and may occasionally justify a trial of low dose steroid e.g. prednisolone 5-7.5mg daily, although results are often disappointing. Arthritis or rashes may respond to such doses but higher doses of steroid should generally be avoided in this type of disease since the risk of toxicty is likely to outweigh benefits. It is important to consider alternative explanations for fatigue such as anaemia, depression, a side-effect of medication or hypothyroidism, which is more common in people with lupus than in the general population. A healthy diet and regular gentle exercise should be encouraged.

NSAIDs are also reasonably effective for symptom control but should be used with caution in lupus as they often cause an increase in blood pressure, fluid retention and can impair renal function. Furthermore, it now seems clear that both conventional NSAIDs (apart, perhaps, from naproxen) and the newer COX-2 selective NSAIDs can cause a modest increase in the risk of heart attack and stroke. As the risk of cardiovascular disease is increased in lupus, any additional risk is to be avoided. They can also impair ovulation and, if used during pregnancy beyond the 20th week, can constrict the ductus arteriosus and impair foetal renal function.

Intermediate disease

This category includes those with pleurisy, pericarditis, severe rashes and haematological manifestations such as thrombocytopenia and leucopenia. In such cases steroids are usually required. The aim is to use a dose sufficient to control the disease and then reduce it to as low a maintenance dose as possible. It is difficult to generalise regarding dose. Pleurisy can usually be controlled by about 20mg prednisolone daily, whereas, haematological problems may require doses of 40mg or more for disease suppression.

Hydroxychloroquine may be adequate in conjunction with steroids but often immunosuppression is required. Azathioprine has been used most widely but in recent years methotrexate has been used increasingly as has mycophenolate. Cyclosporin can also be useful, particularly in the treatment of thrombocytopenia, but because of its tendency to cause hypertension and to impair renal function it has to be used with great care in lupus. All of these drugs take some time to take effect, e.g. 1-3 months, and during this period steroids will be required in a dose sufficient to control the disease. Once the patient is stabilised on the immunosuppressive drug every effort should be made to reduce the dose of steroid to the lowest at which disease control can be maintained.

Severe disease

Significant renal, CNS and severe skin or haematological disease fall into this category. The different sub-types and their distinct prognoses and treatments are discussed in more detail in the relevant chapters. In CNS disease, cerebral lupus has to be distinguished from clotting problems associated with antiphospholipid antibodies, as anticoagulation rather than immunosuppression will be required for the latter. Steroids will almost inevitably be required plus an immunosuppressive drug. Predisolone 1-2mg/kg or pulsed intravenous methylprednisolone may be needed to bring the disease under control. Hydroxychloroquine is rarely adequate in this type of disease. Azathioprine, methotrexate or mycophenolate may be useful for their immunosuppressive and steroid-sparing effects. Treatment can be divided into an initial induction phase in which active disease is brought under control, followed by a maintenance phase of less intensive therapy designed to keep it under control.

Cyclophosphamide has been the mainstay of treatment for severe manifestations of lupus since the landmark NIH trials of the 1980s, especially for bad renal or CNS disease or pneumonitis. This can be given either as intermittent intravenous bolus infusions or taken daily by mouth. The dose and frequency used will depend upon the severity of disease e.g. acute cerebral vasculitis may require weekly intravenous cyclophosphamide plus pulsed intravenous steroid whereas subacute disease such as deteriorating renal function may respond to monthly intravenous or oral cyclophosphamide plus oral steroids. Mycophenolate is proving to be a less toxic and useful alternative to cyclophosphamide and has supplanted it in moderately severe cases, although cyclophosphamide may still have a place in the induction phase of treatment in very severe disease. If cyclophosphamide is used one generally tries to transfer to mycophenolate, azathioprine or methotrexate for maintenance treatment as soon as possible.

Additional treatments used in severe lupus include intravenous immunoglobulin, plasma exchange and monoclonal antibodies. Intravenous immunoglobulin is widely used for thrombocytopenia but can be helpful for other manifestations. Plasma exchange is used less frequently now than in the past but many still believe that it can be helpful in acute, severe disease, particularly cerebral lupus. Monoclonal antibodies, particularly rituximab, are extremely promising and are likely to play a major part in the management of severe and intermediate disease.

Co-morbidity

It has become clear in recent years that lupus is a major risk factor for the development of cardiovascular disease and that myocardial infarction and stroke are much more common in people with lupus than in the general population. As well as conventional risk factors such as hypertension, hyperlipidaemia, smoking and obesity, other factors are involved. These include antiphospholipid antibodies; endothelial dysfunction and lipid peroxidation in the vessel wall; use of NSAIDs and HRT, and steroid-induced diabetes. As well as seeking optimal control of the disease, it is imperative to check blood pressure and fasting lipids and glucose regularly, to institute appropriate treatment where necessary and to strongly discourage smoking in order to minimise cardiovascular risk factors.

Comments on individual drugs

Steroids

The correct use of steroids is key to the management of lupus. The disease may be under-treated but a more common mistake is to continue high dose steroids for too long. Mild disease may respond to 5-10mg prednisolone daily. For more severe disease 20-40mg may be required and for severe disease 1mg/kg or more or the use of pulsed intravenous methylprednisolone. Every effort should be made to taper the dose to the lowest sufficient to maintain disease control. In patients who have had severe disease there is often a flare-up when the daily prednisolone dose is reduced to between 7.5 and 15mg daily. This should be borne in mind when monitoring someone with lupus and it is often wise to reduce the prednisolone by 1mg at a time when the daily dose is below 15mg.

Steroid-induced osteoporosis is a common problem in people with lupus. National guidelines recommend that anyone who receives more than 7.5mg prednisolone daily for three months and is aged 65+ or has had a previous fragility fracture should receive osteoprotective treatment. Younger people should have their bone density measured serially by DEXA scan. We now have effective osteoprotective agents in the form of bisphosphonates (Fosamax, Actonel, Bonviva) and strontium ranelate (Protelos). HRT is no longer used for the prevention or treatment of osteoporosis because of the increased risk of breast cancer and cardiovascular disease. Although Raloxifene (Evista) reduces the risk of breast cancer it increases the risk of venous thromboembolism and has not been shown to reduce the frequency of non-vertebral fractures, so it is a poor alternative to bisphosphonates and strontium ranelate. It is not known whether treatment of women of child-bearing age with bisphosphonates poses any hazard to children born subsequently. Bisphposphonates are contra-indicated during pregnancy and it is recommended that pregnancy should be postponed for six months after withdrawal of bisphosphonates.

Increased susceptibility to infection is another major concern, especially in those who are also on immunosuppressive drugs. Steroids may aggravate hypertension, provoke diabetes and have an adverse effect on lipid profile which probably contributes to the increased cardiovascular mortality in lupus. In high doses steroids increase the risk of gastrointestinal bleeding and will do so at lower doses when taken with NSAIDs. Osteonecrosis (avascular necrosis) is also fairly common in lupus and seems to be associated particularly with the use of high-dose oral steroids or pulsed intravenous methylprednisolone.

Antimalarials

Hydroxychloroquine (Plaquenil) is generally preferred to chloroquine because the risk of ocular toxicity is believed to be greater with the latter. Ocular toxicity is related both to the daily and cumulative dose and the daily dose should not exceed 6.5mg/kg lean body weight. So long as this dose is not exceeded the risk of eye problems is very small. The manufacturers recommend a baseline ophthalmological check and annual review, however, the Royal College of Ophthalmologists has recommended that patients should have baseline and annual visual acuity checks performed by the prescribing doctor and be referred to an ophthalmologist only if a visual problem is identified at baseline or reduced acuity or blurred vision develop on treatment. Hydroxychloroquine has the benefits of reducing cholesterol levels, a modest anti-platelet effect and it may reduce the extent of permanent tissue injury in lupus. Hydroxychloroquine appears to be safe in pregnancy.

The addition of mepacrine 50-100mg daily may be useful in those not responding to hydroxychloroquine alone. Mepacrine is not thought to be associated with ocular side-effects.

Azathioprine

Azathioprine (Imuran) is an immunosuppressant antimetabolite: it reduces purine biosynthesis which is necessary for proliferation of cells including those of the immune system. It is generally used in a dose of 1-2.5mg/kg. Nausea is common while leucopenia and thrombocytopenia occur in some 4% of cases. Monitoring the drug can be a problem if people with lupus already have such clinical features. Abnormal liver function tests occur in a similar proportion of people.

147

Azathiorpine is catabolised by the enzyme thiopurine methyltransferase (TPMT) and about 1 in 300 people have a deficient genetic polymorphism of TPMT which renders them susceptible to severe drug toxicity. Laboratory testing can identify people at risk and so protect them from exposure to the drug, access to such testing is becoming more available in the NHS. Azathioprine is considered safe to use during pregnancy in doses up to 2mg/kg.

Mycophenolate mofetil

Mycophenolate mofetil (CellCept) inhibits purine synthesis, lymphocyte proliferation and T cell-dependent antibody responses. Compared with cyclophosphamide it does not cause ovarian failure and is less likely to be associated with serious infection, leucopenia or severe alopecia. It is also probably more effective and better tolerated than azathioprine. It has rapidly assumed a central role in the management of lupus. It is contra-indicated in pregnancy and should only be used in women of child-bearing age in conjunction with reliable contraception. Because of its long half-life it should be stopped at least six weeks before planned conception.

Methotrexate

Methotrexate (Maxtrex) is a folic acid antagonist and is classified as an antimetabolite cytotoxic agent; it has many effects on cells of the immune system including modulation of cytokine production. It is used in a once weekly regimen typically starting at a dose of 7.5mg per week building up to 20mg weekly if required. Folic acid 5-10mg once weekly (not on the same day as the methotrexate) is routinely given to reduce the risk of side-effects. Nausea and mouth ulcers are fairly common and leucopenia, thrombocytopenia and abnormal liver function tests occur occasionally. Methotrexate is contra-indicated during pregnancy and should be used in women of child-bearing age only in conjunction with effective contraception. The drug should be withdrawn three months before conception is attempted.

Cyclosporin

Cyclosporin (Neoral) inhibits the action of calcineurin and so leads to reduced function of effector T lymphocytes. It is used in a dose of 2.5-5mg/kg daily. Hypertension and an increase in serum creatinine are common and this makes it difficult to use in lupus where such features are often already present. Careful monitoring of blood pressure and creatinine are essential. It is considered reasonable to use it during pregnancy at the lowest effective dose with careful attention to blood pressure and renal function.

Cyclophosphamide

This is an alkylating anti-neoplastic agent. It has been used extensively for the treatment of patients with lupus and internal organ involvement over the past four decades. It has been shown to improve the outcome of renal disease to a greater extent than steroids alone and is still widely used for the treatment of severe CNS, renal or pulmonary disease. It can be given in a daily oral dose of 0.5-2mg/kg, or as intravenous infusions. The dose and frequency of intravenous infusions vary according to disease severity, but doses of 7.5-15mg/kg every four weeks are often used.

The main hazards are increased risk of infection; ovarian failure; bladder toxicity, and increased risk of subsequent malignancy. The risk of haemorrhagic cystitis can be reduced somewhat by giving MESNA concurrently. It is teratogenic and impairs gonadal function in both men and women. Ovarian failure is closely related to the dose given and also the age of the patient: over 25 the risk increases significantly. In young people who want children subsequently storage of sperm or ovarian harvest and storage of eggs should be considered. The drug should be withdrawn three months before conception is attempted.

Intravenous immunoglobulin

This is a recognised treatment for thrombocytopenic purpura and can be helpful for other manifestations of lupus. The mode of action is unclear but saturation of Fc receptors and alteration of the idiotypic network are possible mechanisms. It is usually given in a dose of about 0.5g/kg as an intravenous infusion on three consecutive days and repeated at intervals depending on response. It can be used safely during pregnancy.

Rituximab

Rituximab (Mabthera) is a monoclonal antibody which reacts with the CD20 molecule on mature B cells and pre-B cells. CD20 is not, however, expressed on B cell progenitors or plasma cells, which means that the humoral immune system is not switched off completely. In early studies it was given in combination with cyclophosphamide but now it is often given with methotrexate. Following infusion of rituximab there is a sustained decrease in circulating B cells for several months but only a modest reduction in total immunoglobulin levels. Autoantibody levels tend to fall more than other antibodies. Rituximab has led to dramatic improvement in some people with refractory lupus and a repeat course of treatment has been effective in some of those who relapsed. This agent is being studied in people with earlier disease and clearly represents a major therapeutic advance. Epratuximab, a monoclonal antibody which reacts with another B cell antigen (CD22), is also showing considerable promise.

Other agents

In certain circumstances, other drugs may be needed to control specific disease manifestations, or when more commonly used drugs prove ineffective or are not tolerated. These include mepacrine, leflunomide, dapsone, thalidomide, quinacrine and clofazimine. These are discussed elsewhere in this book. A number of monoclonal antibodies and other biological agents which affect cells of the immune system or inhibit cytokines are being studied and it is very likely that additional agents will become available for treatment within the next few years.

Conclusion

The management of lupus requires careful disease monitoring and interpretation of laboratory results and judicious use of the available drugs. It involves a constant struggle to strike the correct balance between under-treatment and over-treatment of the disease. Patients are often well informed about their disease and should be viewed as partners in disease management. Close collaboration between GP and specialist is essential for optimal disease management.

Table 1. Questions to ask in the management of Lupus

What are the disease manifestations?
How active is the disease?
How am I monitoring the disease?
Am I treating the disease vigorously enough?
Am I overtreating the disease at present?
Am I checking for co-morbidity?
Do I need to involve a colleague?

Remember
Check the blood pressure & renal function regularly
Check the urine for protein regularly
Check fasting lipids & glucose periodically
If uncertain about blood results, disease activity or its management do not hesitate to discuss with a specialist

---

Table 2. Side-effects of drugs and important interactions*

	Very common >10%	Common 1-10%	Uncommon 0.1-1%	Important interactions
Azathioprine	Leucopenia	Thrombocytopenia	Infections Anaemia Pancreatitis	Allopurinol
Cyclosporin	Hypertension Renal dysfunction Tremor Headache Hyperlipidaemia	Nausea Gingival hyperplasia Myalgia Hypertrichosis Paraesthesia Hyperuricaemia	Anaemia Thrombocytopenia	Carbamazepine Phenytoin Erythromycin Diltiazem St John's wort Grapefruit juice
Cyclophosphamide	Leucopenia Azospermia, ovarian failure Alopecia Mouth ulcers	Haemorrhagis cystitis Hyponatraemia	Tumours	Oral hypoglycaemic drugs
Hydroxychloroquine		Nausea Rash	Retinopathy	Digoxin
Methotrexate	Nausea	Mouth ulcers Leucopenia Hepatic dysfunction Diarrhoea	Pneumonitis	Trimethoprim Cotrimoxazole Acitretin
Mycophenolate	Infection Leucopenia Thrombocytopenia Nausea, diarrhoea	Hyperlipidaemia Headache Rash Hepatic & renal dysfunction	Skin cancer	Colestyramine

* Monitoring guidelines can be found on the British Society for Rheumatology website at www.rheumatology.org.uk

Dr Robin Butler, Consultant Rheumatologist
Leopold Muller Arthritis Research Centre
Robert Jones & Agnes Hunt Orthopaedic Hospital
Oswestry, Shropshire SY10 7AG

Alternative and Complementary Medicine in the Treatment of Lupus

Introduction

In most of the world, alternative, or complementary, medicine is widely accepted and in the United Kingdom there is a growing interest in its use. It is thought that almost four billion people globally use plants as medicines, predominantly because nothing else is either affordable or accessible. Estimates worldwide suggest that less than 30% of health care is provided by allopathic (Western-style) medicine. The American College of Rheumatology statement on 'complementary' and 'alternative' therapies for rheumatic disease defines such therapies as 'being outside of the prevailing mainstream and may be safe and effective, unsafe and ineffective or questionable'. It is important to emphasise that 'alternative' medicine is frequently called 'complementary' medicine because the majority of Western patients use this therapy along with, not instead of, allopathic medical care. In the United Kingdom, it is estimated that 20% of the general population visit alternative care practitioners. In the chronic rheumatic diseases, the use of alternative medical therapies is higher than in the general population and ranges from 40-94%. A study published in 2000 showed that nearly 50% of British lupus patients had used alternative medical therapies, the most popular forms being relaxation techniques, massage and herbal medicine (Table 1).

Whilst it is apparent that a large number of patients are using alternative and complementary treatments, the reasons for this are less clear. One explanation for this health seeking behaviour in Western patients is not secondary to a disillusionment with conventional allopathic medicine but, rather, a result of patients' perceptions of a lack of holistic care shown by their medical practitioners. This hypothesis is supported by the fact that in America, where the data is available, over 70% of patients using alternative care are unlikely to disclose this potentially vital information to their regular physicians. The major reason reported for not sharing this information is the belief that mainstream doctors disapprove of alternative therapies and may even refuse to treat them once they discover that their patients are using complementary therapies. Another study suggests that the widespread use of alternative therapies is because allopathic medicine is simply 'unable to comprehensively treat chronic illness' whereas, in addressing the connection between mind and body, complementary medicine can fill a void left by allopathic medicine.

The scope of alternative therapies is vast, and ever increasing. More than 350 practices have been described and in the year 2000 the Food and Drug Administration (FDA) of America estimated that there are more than 29,000 herbal, vitamin or supplement therapies available with approximately 1000 more

152

added each month. In order to provide a structure for this chapter, the various alternative and complementary therapies have been sub-divided according to their classification as defined by the American National Institute of Health. The classification system and sub-grouping of treatment modalities which are covered in this chapter, are found in Table 2.

The aim of this chapter is to serve as a reference in exploring the evidence both for, and against, the principal alternative and complementary therapies used in the treatment of lupus. As a quick guide, at the end of each section there is a brief summary of the preceding evidence.

Table 1 - The use of alternative medical therapies by lupus patients in the United Kingdom, Canada and the United States. The total refers to all patients using at least one alternative therapy and the numbers in brackets are the percentage (%) of patients in that category.

	United Kingdom (n=211)	Canada (n=229)	United States (n=267)
Relaxation techniques	45 (21.3)	51 (22.3)	71 (26.6)
Massage	40 (19)	36 (15.7)	52 (19.5)
Herbal Medicine	32 (15.2)	28 (12.2)	28 (10.5)
Lifestyle diets	27 (12.8)	26 (11.4)	41 (15.4)
Spiritual healing	14 (6.6)	16 (7)	39 (14.6)
Commercial weight loss	14 (6.6)	8 (3.5)	18 (6.7)
Homeopathy	13 (6.2)	14 (6.1)	6 (2.2)
Megavitamin therapy	10 (4.7)	14 (6.1)	14 (5.2)
Self-help groups	10 (4.7)	21 (9.2)	29 (10.9)
Acupuncture	8 (3.8)	7 (3.1)	3 (1.1)
Imagery	7 (3.3)	18 (7.9)	26 (9.7)
Energy healing	6 (2.8)	11 (4.8)	6 (2.2)
Folk remedies	4 (1.9)	18 (7.9)	10 (3.7)
Chiropractic	4 (1.9)	15 (6.6)	13 (4.9)
Hypnosis	3 (1.4)	3 (1.3)	3 (1.1)
Biofeedback	0 (0)	8 (3.5)	10 (3.7)
Other	13 (6.2)	10 (4.4)	8 (3)
Total	**102 (48.3)**	**116 (50.7)**	**134 (50.2)**

Table 2 - Classification of Alternative Modalities and Therapies.

Fields of Practice – ANIH	Alternative Modalities/Therapies	Examples covered in this chapter
Diet, nutrition and lifestyle changes	Promotes study of effects of foods, vitamins and minerals on acute and chronic disease, with additional focus on health maintenance and disease prevention.	Essential fatty acids Vitamins A and E Selenium Evening Primrose Oil Green tea products Food elimination diets
Herbal Medicine	Includes herbal products for pharmacological use; derived from European, Asian and Native American traditions.	Uncaria tomentosa Uncaria guianensis (cats claw)
Mind/body interventions and movement therapies	Includes therapies such as biofeedback, relaxation, imagery, meditation, hypnosis, psychotherapy, prayer, dance, music therapy and yoga.	Meditation Hypnosis Cognitive behavioural therapy Exercise Aromatherapy
Alternative systems of medical practice	Consists of traditional Oriental medicine.	Acupuncture Moxibustion
Manual healing methods	Uses techniques such as osteopathy, massage, chiropractic, and thera-peutic touch as diagnostic and therapeutic tools.	Massage Reflexology
Bioelectromagnetics	Explores the interaction of living organisms with electromagnetic fields for multiple healthcare applications	Electro-magnetic field devices
Pharmacological and biological Interventions	Includes drugs and vaccines not yet endorsed by mainstream medical practice.	Diet

1.0 Diet and Nutritional Therapies

Attempts at symptom management can often leave patients feeling totally dominated by their disease. In their quest to regain some control, and with dietary modification and 'fad diets' becoming more frequently promoted to the general public, a number of patients try dietary modification and supplements with varying success. The following section outlines a number of diet and nutritional therapies, their benefits and potential deleterious effects.

1.1 Essential Fatty Acids

The role of essential fatty acids and dietary oils has been investigated with the omega-3 polyunsaturated fatty acids derived from fish oils being shown to have effective immunomodulatory activities.

Studies in humans have shown that prolonged treatment with omega-3 fatty acids in the form of fish oils can slow renal progression for high-risk patients with IgA nephropathy and lower plasma triglycerides, but it must be noted that these studies have small numbers. Other research has suggested that in patients who already exhibit disease, an increased consumption of omega-3 fatty acids is not necessarily beneficial, but it could potentially prevent relapse. In a number of randomized controlled clinical trials of rheumatoid arthritis, the use of omega-3 fatty acids has been shown to be beneficial and reduce NSAID requirements. Similarly, whilst the results of trials using fatty acids in patients with inflammatory bowel disease are variable, a number of studies have shown a significant benefit to both clinical activity and steroid-sparing effect.

Further research has also investigated the use of flaxseed oil (also known as linseed oil) in patients with lupus nephritis. Flaxseed contains high concentrations of the omega-3 fatty acid precursor a-linolenic acid and it is this which is thought to produce the beneficial effects. Results in humans indicate that flaxseed appears to be renoprotective in lupus nephritis and can reduce serum creatinine and improve creatinine clearance. However, these results should be interpreted with caution given the small numbers of patients in the trials.

Whilst there are some positive studies using fatty acids in humans with lupus, there is clearly the need for further carefully designed controlled trials into their therapeutic application in human autoimmune and inflammatory conditions. Before this research is available, there is no harm (unless the patient has an allergy) in patients increasing their intake of omega-3 fatty acids by using oils rich in these fatty acids and increasing their intake of oily fish to two to three times per week.

1.2 Vitamins A and E

Vitamin A products (retinoids) are already extensively used by dermatologists in the treatment of psoriasis and acne. Research in three women given vitamin A (beta-carotene) three times a day in 1976 showed a clearing of skin lesions within one week of commencing treatment. A further study of 10 women in 1988 showed beneficial responses to high doses of supplementary vitamin A given for two weeks. Whilst these studies showed no side effects of vitamin A, there is a lack of research into the long-term effects of Vitamin A and its impact. It is known that the ingestion of excess vitamin A from animal sources can have side effects including alopecia, nausea and anorexia and, therefore, at present it can only be recommended that patients have a balanced diet containing sufficient plant-based Vitamin A, e.g. from carrots and sweet potatoes.

Studies on lupus mice models have shown that treatment with vitamin E can delay the onset of autoimmunity and extend mean survival time. However, these findings have not been satisfactorily replicated in humans and treating lupus with vitamin E is still controversial, despite research into the topic first being available in the 1940's. A more recent study looking at disease activity in 12 patients through recording oxidative DNA damage and autoantibodies suggests that vitamin E can be of benefit but older studies of vitamin E in the treatment of discoid skin lesions have given variable outcomes. There are some anxieties that vitamin E is only effective in the treatment of lupus at very high doses but that, even at high doses, patients still appear to have flares and that at these doses vitamin E can function as an anticoagulant. There is, therefore, a need for further research to investigate the clinical effectiveness of this vitamin in lupus patients, both as to its effects on skin lesions and on total disease activity.

1.3 Selenium

Free radical damage is known to play a significant role in the pathogenesis of lupus and research has shown that there are low levels of antioxidants in the serum of lupus patients. A number of studies have suggested that antioxidant supplementation may improve lupus disease activity. Selenium is a natural antioxidant. It appears that the supplementation of auto-immune mice models with selenium results in increased life expectancy and a significantly higher level of natural killer cell activity. The mechanisms behind these findings are not known. Dietary sources with high levels of selenium include fish such as pike, carp and herring. However, it must be noted that excess selenium can result in toxicity which may present with symptoms such as alopecia, gastrointestinal disturbance, sloughing of the nails and, in extreme cases, liver cirrhosis, pulmonary oedema and death. Patients must, therefore, be warned against taking excessive selenium supplementation.

1.4 Evening Primrose Oil

Research has shown that evening primrose oil supplementation can increase survival in autoimmune mice models. It is thought that this effect results from an increase in prostaglandin E_1, and that the prostaglandin is derived from gamma-linolenic acid which constitutes 19% of the content of evening primrose oil. Prostaglandin E_1 is thought to exert its beneficial activities in lupus models through decreasing lymphocyte proliferation and natural killer cell activity. These studies have not been replicated in humans and, therefore, evening primrose oil cannot be routinely recommended.

1.5 Green Tea Products

Epidemiological evidence indicates that in comparison to the United States and Britain, the incidence of lupus is considerably lower in China and Japan, the two leading green-tea consuming countries. It is hypothesized that green tea polyphenols (GTPs) may be at least partly responsible for this geographical difference in lupus severity and prevalence. To support this theory, a number of molecular, cellular and animal studies have indicated that GTPs can provide protective effects against autoimmune reactions in salivary glands (particularly important in Sjögren's Syndrome) and in the skin by suppressing autoantigen expression and down-regulating inflammatory cytokines. These studies have not been replicated in humans but preliminary data appears promising. Further research would be needed to check out any beneficial effects of GTPs.

1.6 Dietary Considerations and Food Elimination Diets

Much of the research previously covered concerns diet modification and the potential inclusion of high vitamin, anti-oxidant or nutrient foods. The following section outlines a number of diet modifications which may help ameliorate lupus symptoms/signs.

1.6.1 Alfalfa Seeds

Alfalfa is primarily used in the United States, Australia and New Zealand for dairy production, beef and lamb. However, it is also used for human consumption, particularly as a salad ingredient in these countries. Over the past few decades there has been interest and research into alfalfa's cholesterol lowering activities. Interestingly, researchers observed pancytopaenia and antinuclear antibody production in both primates and humans who were given alfalfa seeds and, in primates, symptoms such as lethargy, anorexia and a facial rash which resolved when the treatment was withdrawn and were exacerbated again on re-introduction of alfalfa seeds.

Further research examining the link between alfalfa and lupus concluded that the amino acid L-canavanine was the key constituent of alfalfa which exacerbated lupus, though a lack of control over autoantibody synthesis and lymphocyte proliferation. L-canavanine is found in many legumes including soyabean, alfalfa, clover and onions, however, cooking the food is meant to destroy the lupus-provoking effects whilst maintaining lipid-lowering properties. Therefore, it is recommended that lupus patients avoid alfalfa and cook foods which are rich in L-canavanine.

1.6.2 Excess Energy, Protein and Fat

A number of animal studies suggest that energy and calorie restriction reduces autoimmune disease. However, whilst it is known that lupus disease activity is associated with an increase in body mass index in pre-menopausal women, there do not appear to be any studies into caloric restriction in humans and the effects this has on lupus activity. Such studies would be impossible to directly repeat in humans given that in animal models scientists have reduced caloric intake by up to 60% in pre-adolescent mice.

High protein intake is known to be associated with an acceleration of kidney disease in both autoimmune-prone individuals and animal models and, therefore, it is widely accepted that low protein diets are the standard treatment for renal failure. The benefits of omega-3 polyunsaturated fatty acids in lupus have previously been outlined. Saturated or omega-6 polyunsaturated fats have been shown to have a detrimental effect on autoimmune disease activity and reduce survival in a number of animal models. Autoimmune-prone mice fed saturated fats appear to experience more severe nephritis and glomerular pathology, leading to the hypothesis that dietary fat, especially saturated fat, restriction may be an effective therapeutic approach to lupus nephritis. Research in humans is sparse, but one study followed patients with lupus who reduced their intake of omega-6 polyunsaturated fats for one year. In this study, the number of patients with active disease fell from 11 to 3 but the study group was small, there was no control group and there was the additional possibility of spontaneous improvement and a placebo effect. Foods high in omega-6 fatty acids include oils such as sunflower oil, poppy seed oil, corn oil and foods such as mayonnaise, margarine and brazil nuts.

In addition to generic reduction diets of calories, fats and protein, a number of researchers have suggested that lupus patients may be more likely to have food allergies. A number of case studies indicate that lupus patients may benefit from the discovery and elimination of possible food triggers.

Summary

- Omega-3 fatty acids from fish oils (oily fish) and flaxseed oil (linseed oil) can, possibly, slow renal progression in lupus patients. Patients can be encouraged to increase their intake of omega-3 fatty acids to two or three times per week, unless they have an allergy.
- Vitamin A can help reduce lupus skin lesions. Long term effects of vitamin A are not known but patients should be encouraged to eat a balanced diet with sufficient plant based Vitamin A (good sources being carrots and sweet potatoes).

- The evidence regarding vitamin E and lupus is equivocal but, again, a balanced diet is advocated.
- Selenium (a natural antioxidant found in fish such as pike, carp and herring) may improve disease activity. Supplementation should not be excessive as this may lead to toxicity.
- The evidence regarding evening primrose oil in lupus is equivocal.
- The evidence regarding green tea products is equivocal, but patients should not be discouraged from drinking moderate amounts.
- As there is no harm in doing so, it is recommended that patients avoid alfalfa and cook foods rich in L-canavanine (onions, soya bean).
- There is currently insufficient evidence, but some research indicates that a low protein diet and reduction in consumption of foods rich in omega-6 polyunsaturated fats (e.g. sunflower oil, mayonnaise) may be beneficial in lupus patients.

2.0 Herbal Treatments

With the 'natural products' field growing at an increasing rate, both patients and healthcare workers need reliable information in order to make appropriate treatment choices. Patients may well have started taking herbal remedies on the subjective advice of enthusiastic but uninformed sales staff. Many sales suggestions come from anecdotal or personal experience and this can put patients at risk. Herbal products are classified as dietary supplements and the normal regulatory controls for medicines do not apply. The lack of regulation over herbal treatments is important both because as single agents the 'natural products' can cause toxicity and side-effects but also because they may interact in unexpected ways with other prescribed medication, particularly disease modifying anti-rheumatic drugs (DMARDs) such as methotrexate and mycophenolate. Therefore, if patients express an interest in herbal remedies, a qualified medical specialist should be consulted before any are taken.

2.1 Uncaria tomentosa and Uncaria guianensis

Uncaria tomentosa and Uncaria guianensis are Peruvian herbs commonly known as 'cat's claw'. Traditionally, the bark of 'cat's claw' is prepared as a decoction (water which the plant has previously been boiled in) which is said to be beneficial in the treatment of arthritis, bursitis, chronic fatigue syndrome and disorders of the gastrointestinal tract as well as lupus. The mechanism of action of these two herbs is not currently known, but it is thought that perhaps U. tomentosa functions through inhibition of TNFa production. Whilst there are no animal or human trials of either of these herbs in lupus patients, there is a 52-week double blind placebo-controlled study of 40 patients with active rheumatoid arthritis who were randomized to U. tomentosa or placebo in addition to their standard treatment with sulfasalazine or hydroxychloroquine. Results showed a 53%

reduction in the number of painful joints in patients receiving the *U. tomentosa*, in comparison to a 24% reduction in the placebo group. As a note of caution, there is one reported case of acute renal failure secondary to treatment with 'cat's claw' in a patient who had lupus.

2.2 Other Herbal Remedies

A number of other herbs have also been investigated in lupus mice with the hope of reducing the necessity for steroids. *Atractylodes ovata, Angelica sinensis, Cordyceps sinensis, Ligustrum ludidum* and *Codonopsis pilosula* extracts were all tested, the most effective being *C. sinensis* which exhibited the greatest inhibition of anti double-stranded DNA antibodies and longest lifespan of affected mice. The mechanism of action of these remedies is not yet known. One human study of 61 lupus patients given *C.sinensis* over five years showed a slower deterioration in creatinine clearance, however, more research, human models and greater validation is needed.

Summary

- Natural remedies are not subjected to the same rigorous testing and licensing laws as drugs and, therefore, can have potentially serious and poorly documented side effects.
- Herbal remedies should not be used without specialist advice, particularly if patients are also taking DMARDs.

3.0 Mind/Body Interventions and Movement Therapies

The idea that the mind can influence the body and vice versa is not a new concept, for example, in clinical trials, the 'placebo effect' is well known. However, there is now an increasing body of evidence to support the psychoneuroimmunology theory which provides a conceptual framework for the brain's ability to control all aspects of the immune system. If this connection between mind and body is accepted, then this can provide a key to treatment. The major categories of 'mind/body' treatments are outlined below.

3.1 Meditation

Meditation has its foundation in early religious practices and over the past few decades it has become more widely accepted as a treatment for chronic illness. In practicing meditation, individuals use particular awareness and concentration techniques to calm the mind and relax the body. There is no specific research into meditation in lupus, however, research in patients with fibromyalgia has shown that meditation can help relieve pain, anxiety, stress, depression and fatigue. Meditation instructors are not certified or licensed on a national level and it is, therefore, important that patients enquire about the training and qualifications of any individuals or organizations they wish to approach for care. Before meditation can be widely recommended further research is needed to validate its therapeutic potential.

3.2 Hypnosis

Hypnotherapy involves bringing a patient into a state where they are unaware of, but not blind to, their surroundings and they are in a state of focused and attentive concentration. Hypnotherapy has been studied as a tool for managing a variety of problems including chronic pain syndromes, irritable bowel, fibromyalgia and arthritis. There is one case report where hypnotherapy was used in conjunction with psychoanalytic psychotherapy to help a young female with lupus and there is a paper suggesting a protocol for use in hypnosis in patients with a variety of complaints, including lupus, but there does not appear to be any other published research in the therapeutic benefits of hypnosis specifically in lupus.

3.3 Cognitive Behavioural Therapy and Stress Reduction

Cognitive behavioural therapy is a multidisciplinary approach which involves teaching patients new thought and behaviour patterns for coping with chronic illness. A randomized controlled trial of a stress-reduction program using biofeedback-assisted cognitive-behavioural therapy in 92 patients who experienced pain with lupus found that patients who received the treatment showed improvements in pain, psychological function and perceived physical function. Although the study number was relatively small, these results are promising and, potentially, could offer a helpful intervention to reduce pain without additional medication. However, the treatment requires several clinic visits with a trained health professional and this is not only time consuming for the patient but could present funding issues.

Slightly different options which have been researched in lupus patients include self-help groups which are reported to improve depression, self-worth and self efficacy, or a person-centred telephone counselling system which can improve perceived physical functioning but not pain or psychological functioning.

3.4 Exercise

A recent review which focused on the relationship between lupus and exercise in patients with low to moderate disease activity, found that exercise can help patients with lupus in a number of ways. Exercise can help reduce cardiovascular mortality, obesity, osteoporosis, sleep disturbances, fatigue and improve quality of life. The authors advise that in order to avoid risks of exercise which come from a wide variation in resting heart rate and blood pressure in lupus patients, individuals should have exercise programs tailored to their personal needs. A major problem in suggesting to patients with chronic disease that they should participate in physical exercise is a lack of adherence and this is particularly the case if patients are exercising individually. Therefore, any exercise programs need to include motivating factors.

Whilst there is no specific evidence regarding Tai Chi or Yoga in lupus patients, these complementary therapies may be of benefit as they encourage patients to 'increase levels of fitness and flexibility within his/her own limits'. It should be noted that, as with all the previously mentioned therapies, patients are advised to learn Tai Chi or Yoga from a teacher rather than simply a video or guidebook.

3.5 Aromatherapy

Aromatherapy is based around essential plant oils and their healing properties. Natural oils are diluted in a carrier oil and normally massaged into the body but they can also be inhaled or used in a cold compress or in a bath. Aromatherapy massages use techniques to relieve tension and improve circulation, the aim being to allow oil molecules to be absorbed into the bloodstream and pass through to the nervous system. There are no trials of aromatherapy in lupus patients, however, there is a paper which suggests that in rheumatoid and musculoskeletal autoimmune disorders aromatherapy is often of value, even if all it serves to do is relax the patient.

Summary

- Psychoneuroimmunology theories suggest that the brain can control all aspects of the immune system.
- The bulk of published information concerning mind/body interventions promotes cognitive behavioural therapy as helping to reduce pain and stress. Aromatherapy, hypnosis and meditation have additionally been promoted as treatment.
- Whilst rarely detrimental, psychological interventions are time consuming and there is a sparsity of information regarding cost effectiveness.
- Exercise should be promoted in patients with mild to moderate disease activity. Tailored exercise programs which include motivating factors are of particular benefit.
- Tai Chi or Yoga can be regarded as forms of exercise and stress reduction. Patients should be encouraged to attend professional training centres rather than teach themselves these techniques.

4.0 Alternative Systems of Medical Practice

Acupuncture is a technique which has been used as pain relief in traditional Chinese medicine for centuries. Acupuncture involves the insertion of fine needles into the skin at a number of specific points along particular channels or meridians. The theory behind acupuncture is that an essential life force flows through the body along these specific channels and that stimulation of these points can correct any misplaced flow and, therefore, reinstate maximum health. Interestingly, whilst some acupuncture points lie in 'trigger points' which are areas rich in nerve endings, a number of meridians do not correspond anatomically to the nervous or circulatory system. There is a lack of large randomized control trial evidence on the efficacy of acupuncture and this is as applicable to lupus as to any other disease. The best evidence using acupuncture is in the treatment of acute pain where it appears to be an effective treatment. There are a number of very small scale trials in patients with lupus, suggesting that acupuncture can possibly reduce the requirement for corticosteroids and help control skin flares in discoid lupus.

Research has also been carried out into moxibustion, another form of traditional Chinese medicine, that uses the heat generated by burning herbal preparations containing Artemisia vulgaris to stimulate acupuncture points. The largest published control study investigated 12 patients with lupus and 12 healthy controls. The study showed no significant alteration in disease activity between the lupus patients and control group. More research is needed to confirm or refute these preliminary findings.

Summary

- There is very little evidence supporting acupuncture therapy for lupus and, therefore, acupuncture cannot be routinely recommended. It may reduce skin flares in discoid lupus but more research is necessary.

5.0 Manual Healing Techniques
5.1 Massage and Reflexology

Despite massage being the second most commonly used alternative/complementary therapy for British lupus patients, there is no published evidence as to its therapeutic benefits in these patients. However, there are a number of studies highlighting the short term benefits of massage in arthritis pain and, for patients with lupus, there is anecdotal evidence that, as with aromatherapy, it can be useful even if all it serves to do is relax the patient.

Reflexology is a particular type of massage that is also widely practiced throughout the world. In reflexology, an individual's feet are viewed as a map of the body with reflexes corresponding to organs or glands. Practitioners promote reflexology on the basis that deals with the principle that there are reflexes in our hands and feet which correspond with every organ, gland and part of the body. Therefore, reflexologists believe that if the reflexes are worked on there will be relief of tension and stress which they consider are the causes of a significant proportion (70%) of today's health problems. This process has not been scientifically validated and there are no studies of reflexology in patients with lupus.

Summary

- Despite a lack of evidence promoting its effectiveness, massage is commonly used by lupus patients.
- Patients should receive massage, chiropractic or reflexology from professionally certified practitioners.

6.0 Bioelectromagnetics

There have been studies investigating the use of pulsed electromagnetic field (EMF) devices in patients with fatigue as a complication of multiple sclerosis. EMF devices deliver low-level, pulsed electromagnetic fields and are worn for up to 24 hours daily on one or more acupressure points for 4 or 8 weeks. Results from two trials have been promising, showing improvement in fatigue levels, particularly in patients with moderate disability levels. However, there was no long term follow up of the patients after either of the trials ended and there do not appear to be any published studies in lupus patients. In spite of this, EMF may be a useful treatment in patients with fatigue as a presenting feature in lupus and this, therefore, warrants further investigation.

Summary

- Pulsed electromagnetic field (EMF) devices may help improve fatigue but more research is needed.

7.0 Other Points of Interest

7.1 Financial Implications of Alternative and Complementary Medicine

As with any treatments, there are cost implications both in the use of complementary medicines and in their evaluation. Two BMJ articles explored the pros and cons of a review by NICE into the effectiveness of alternative and complementary medicine. The principal argument against such an investigation was on financial grounds: 'a strong argument can be made for NICE not having to spend time and money going through, yet again, evidence that we know to be inadequate'. In terms of the actual cost versus benefit of using alternative and complementary medicine, the evidence is not clear but sense would say that any clinically ineffective healthcare is unlikely to be cost-effective. An American study of general medical practice demonstrated that individuals who use complementary medical therapists additionally make more frequent visits to allopathic medical practitioners in comparison to non-users. A Canadian study showed that users of alternative medical therapies made less visits to general practitioners per annum but a similar number of visits to alternative specialists.

7.2 The ethics of alternative therapy

For the practicing clinician, the use of alternative medical therapy can create a number of ethical dilemmas. Physicians have a duty to their patients to respect their autonomy and, therefore, allow freedom of choice as to their desire to seek alternative treatments. However, as previously outlined, there are a number of unanswered questions regarding alternative treatments. Is the conventional approach clearly superior? What is the safety and efficacy of the proposed treatment? Justice could dictate that alternative treatments should be available to all, but at what cost? Nonmaleficence obliges all physicians to make their patients aware of the possible risks but many of the risks are theoretical and treatments may still be beneficial.

Conclusion

This chapter has outlined a number of therapies used in the treatment of specific symptoms in patients affected by lupus. Some treatments have reasonably good evidence for use and appear to be beneficial, even if the mechanism of action is not apparent and, for others, the evidence is less clear.

In order to advise patients about the use of complementary medicines, there are several guidelines that can be referred to, a particularly useful one being published by the department of health. Physicians need to ask their patients about self-medication and complementary or alternative medication and encourage their patients to seek advice from themselves as to any doubts they may have about particular treatments. Physicians should additionally encourage patients to seek licensed practitioners (where available) such as for acupuncture and massage. The department of health provides details of how to contact qualified practitioners. Patients need to know which herbal remedies they are taking, be aware of possible side effects and purchase these from reputable sources with clear labelling. Patients should additionally be encouraged to obtain an accurate diagnosis from a qualified physician before exclusively using alternative treatments for serious conditions with proven conventional treatments.

Despite this chapter highlighting the fact that many alternative therapies need further research in order to determine their efficacy and safety profile, patients will continue to use these treatments regardless of whether this research is performed. Physicians must, therefore, be prepared to counsel and advise patients about all available options with the best available evidence. For an increasing number of patients 'all available options' will mean incorporating alternative medicine into their health care.

Summary

- The evidence for and against complementary and alternative medicine for lupus is mixed and varies with different treatments.
- The department of health has published useful guidelines for complementary medicine.
- It is essential that physicians ask their patients whether they are taking complementary medication and, if patients are keen to seek complementary care, to encourage them to visit qualified practitioners.

Dr Hannah Bainbridge
Royal Sussex County Hospital
Eastern Road
Brighton
East Sussex BN2 5BE

Dr Inam Haq
Brighton & Sussex Medical School
University of Sussex
Brighton
East Sussex BN1 9PX

Physiotherapy

Introduction

Chartered Physiotherapists, those registered with the Health Professions Council UK, are equipped to respond to the needs of lupus patients through effective and appropriate assessment of specific problems identified by individuals. Symptoms vary within and across patients and so it is important to identify the specific concerns, along with a careful consideration of the general features that may be apparent at assessment. Good clinical judgement should lead physiotherapists to determine how they might provide effective management and suitable treatment options based upon best evidence available to them. Therapy and rehabilitation goals should aim at increasing efficiency in activity, with a view to maintaining and improving quality of life.

Management and Treatment

At assessment, clinicians will engage in a two-fold process. They will approach lupus as a multi-system disease affecting many tissues and organ systems whilst evaluating the consequence of these changes on a person's life style and their possible aspirations. A diligent review of these factors will contribute in some measure in proposing physiotherapeutic management and other treatment.

The aim of the physiotherapist in the care of the lupus patient will be to provide:

- Appropriate, ongoing assessment of individuals and management of key clinical features and symptoms
- Propose and agree possible therapeutic strategies with patients
- Consider means for future access and review

It is understood that around 60% of people with lupus describe muscle pain, muscle weakness and tenderness. About 90% have some evidence of arthritis and associated joint problems. These compound the experience of day-to-day living. Faced by such issues, the physiotherapist in discussion with the patient may opt for one, or a combination of the following:

- Management of inflammation and the principles of joint protection
- Pain Management
- Encourage and facilitate efficient movement
- Appropriate exercise prescription
- Consider energy conservation
- Possible ergonomic advice for home, the work place or leisure
- Other coping techniques, stress reduction, relaxation, strategies to assist self
- Education of carers

Physiotherapists have a variety of manual skills and other treatment modalities as part of their therapeutic provision. These will be considered carefully and on an individual basis. They may include exercise prescription, activity to promote efficient movement, improve exercise capacity and encourage good posture and functional movement. Along with this, the use of other modalities that promote pain relief, reduce joint stiffness, reduce muscle discomfort and encourage relaxation will be considered. Typically, therapeutic modalities, including use of electrical equipment and hydrotherapy, can be used to assist pain relief and reduce the effects of inflammation. Complementary therapeutic options, including acupuncture, may be available.

Some of the treatments available include:

- TENS
- Interferential Therapy
- Laser
- Heat
- Hydrotherapy
- Appropriate Manual Therapy

Increasingly, the move within healthcare is to involve patients at every stage of their care and lupus patients should reasonably expect both direct treatment and assistance in developing and appraising self-management skills so they can cope with daily life, demands and choices. Modern healthcare encourages a partnership approach and liaison/consultation with occupational therapists (and other health professionals) may be essential in terms of further specialist advice and expertise. Such items as working/ resting splints and other aids/equipment may be necessary for home and work life, these may be better provided through occupational therapy services.

General Practitioners should consider referring their lupus patients to Physiotherapy Services; these are often available locally within Primary Care Trusts, local rehabilitation day units or health centres.

Finally, changes in government directive regarding health care initiatives and services have led to general programmes becoming available including the Expert Patient Programmes and a course in Challenging Arthritis. In some areas specific clinics and services will be apparent. It is worth investigating what local provision can offer.

Clive Liles
Chartered Physiotherapist
School of Health Sciences
University of Birmingham
Edgbaston B15 2TT

Occupational Therapy

Introduction

Occupational Therapists (OTs) have a number of skills and techniques that can be helpful to people with lupus. They are employed by the NHS and work in OT Departments in District General Hospitals, where they offer both in-patient and out-patient services, as well as in the Community from where they tend to work with people in their own homes. There are also OTs employed by Social Services who are involved in Home Assessments, the provision of equipment and the planning of structural alterations. All these OTs are in touch with each other and provide a network of care for people in need of their services. They can be accessed via Hospital Specialists, General Practitioners or Social Workers. Others work free-lance or for private agencies.

Not every person with lupus will need OT support but specialist advice can be particularly helpful under the following circumstances:

Arthritis

Physiotherapy is often appropriate but OT is particularly helpful where the upper limb is affected, especially the hands and wrists. When the arthritis is acute splints are custom-made to support the joints of the hands and wrists to provide rest and pain relief as well as to hold the joints in optimal positions to prevent the shortening of tendons and ligaments that may result in deformity. The splints may be for night use or for daytime wear to provide support during activity. Whilst Physiotherapists tend to work on muscle power in the bigger muscles, OTs teach exercises to promote the fine movements and tasks performed by the hands. They will also teach a regime of 'joint sparing' in Activities of Daily Living (ADL) to decrease the stress on inflamed joints. The use of thickened grips and handles on utensils, tap levers etc. are examples of these measures.

Aids and Appliances

When there is some degree of physical disability due, for instance, to arthritis, neurological lesions, shortness of breath or extreme fatigue, considerable benefit may be derived from the provision of aids and appliances. A wide variety of these are available through the NHS, Social Services or by private purchase so advice on which are the most suitable is helpful. OTs will carry out an assessment of ADL which includes washing, dressing, toileting, mobility, cooking, hobbies, work tasks etc. and is best done in the home and workplace. Solutions vary from simple gadgets like long-handled shoehorns to adapted keyboards for computer users or 'hands free' telephones. The OT will also give advice on how to apply for equipment that is available from the Statutory Services and on suppliers from whom other items can be purchased.

Mobility Aids

There are a variety of frames and walkers (some folding), perching stools, high seats and sprung cushions for aiding getting up and walking. For people with more severe mobility problems a folding manual wheelchair or an electric-powered wheelchair would facilitate getting about and may well expand activities and widen horizons. Again, there are many different types and it is important for a wheelchair user to have an appropriate model to provide good position and seating and to meet the required range of activities. Some are available through the NHS via the District Wheelchair Service which provides a range of manual and electric powered chairs. A Voucher Scheme has been introduced for people eligible for wheelchairs but perhaps wishing a wider choice. It is usual for OTs to make the referral to the Wheelchair Service.

Home Adaptations

Necessary Home Adaptations may include widening doorways and fitting access ramps to facilitate wheelchair use, lowering kitchen work surfaces, installing showers and fitting lifts or stair lifts. People with severe physical disability may need special mattresses, slings and hoists or, perhaps, a specially designed en-suite bathroom. Sometimes the preferred option would be to move house to ground floor or specially adapted accommodation. These are major and complex issues and the OTs attached to Social Services are expert at assessing needs and solutions and giving advice. Under some circumstances financial help is available and OTs and Social Workers will advise on eligibility and how to apply.

Workplace Adaptations

When someone with a physical disability needs special equipment, structural adaptations or special training to obtain or retain work there may be help available from the Employment Service. In such a case it would often be an OT who would do the initial assessments of need and would then make a referral to the Employment Service via the Disability Employment Adviser based at a Jobcentre.

Dr Sylvia Lachmann FRCP
Lecturer in Rehabilitation Medicine (Retired)
University of Cambridge

Endorsement

Lupus is an important disease and our knowledge and understanding of it has grown rapidly in recent years. It is, therefore, a very good time for LUPUS UK to revise and extend a guide that covers all aspects of the disease in a clear, readable way.

The primary purpose of this guide is to raise awareness of lupus among General Practitioners and Associated Health Professionals with the aim of ensuring early diagnosis and treatment of patients. I am sure it will not only do this but will also make a good text on the subject for patients and their families who are increasingly literate in medicine and the medical sciences.

I congratulate LUPUS UK on undertaking this task and producing the revised guide which I expect to be a great success.

Prof Sir Peter Lachmann FRS FMedSci   National Patron
Emeritus Sheila Joan Smith Professor of Immunology   LUPUS UK
University of Cambridge

LUPUS UK

LUPUS UK is the only national charity caring for people with lupus. 30 Regional Groups cover the UK and over 100 Contacts give support to members and provide advice for those with lupus symptoms who seek knowledge of the illness and possible diagnosis.

The charity offers a comprehensive range of Factsheets and books on lupus and can supply, free of charge, separate Information Packs for individuals, nurses and GPs.

The LUPUS UK national magazine News & Views is published on subscription three times each year and carries regular medical articles on lupus.

LUPUS AWARENESS

Awareness of lupus is an all-year issue where patients, relatives and friends, support groups and others strive to increase understanding of the illness by the general public and medical profession.

LUPUS UK, its Regional Groups and members, also work hard to promote special annual events

OCTOBER
is
LUPUS AWARENESS MONTH

MAY 10th
is
WORLD LUPUS DAY

Publicity materials, leaflets, posters, media releases and more are always available from the charity's National Office to help increase awareness of lupus in clinics, hospitals and public places.

LUPUS UK, St James House, Eastern Road, Romford, Essex, RM1 3NH
Tel: 01708 731251   Fax: 01708 731252
www.lupusuk.org.uk

Further copies of
LUPUS – Diagnosis and Treatment
are available from LUPUS UK
free of charge if requested on GP/clinic/hospital letterheads

Copies are available to others at £6 each inclusive of postage and packing

Further Reading

Lupus – a Guide for Patients	- Prof Graham Hughes	- £3.00 (24pages)
Lupus – Your First 100 Questions	- Prof Graham Hughes	- £3.00 (28 pages)
Hughes Syndrome – a Patient's Guide	- Prof Graham Hughes	- £5.00 (64 pages)
Lupus – Everything You Need to Know	- Dr R Lahita/Dr R Philips	- £10.50 (224 pages)
Coping with Lupus	- Dr R Philips	- £12.50 (383 pages)
The Lupus Book	- Dr Daniel Wallace	- £13.50 (258 pages)
Talking About Lupus	- Triona Holden	- £7.99 (200 pages)
A Patient's Guide to Lupus	- Prof Graham Hughes	- £5.99 (112 pages)
Lupus – The Facts	- Prof David Isenberg/ Prof Susan Manzi	- £9.99 (112 pages)

Please add £1 per book – postage & packing

PATIENT FACTSHEETS

LUPUS the Symptoms & Diagnosis LUPUS the Joints & Muscles
LUPUS and the Kidneys LUPUS the Skin & Hair
LUPUS the Heart & Lungs LUPUS the Mouth, Nose & Eyes
LUPUS and the Brain LUPUS and Blood Disorders
LUPUS and Medication LUPUS and Light Sensitivity
LUPUS and Pregnancy LUPUS and Associated Conditions
LUPUS a Guide for Patients LUPUS Fatigue & Your Lifestyle
LUPUS and Men LUPUS and the Feet
LUPUS Incidence within the Community

PATIENT BOOKLETS

Discoid Lupus
A short Guide to Lupus & Visiting Your Doctor
My Lupus - What I Need to Know - A Young Person's Guide

Factsheets/booklets available free of charge if requested on GP/clinic/hospital letterheads

Available to others: 5 factsheets/booklets free of charge
                        6-10   "   "   £2 donation requested
                        11-15   "   "   £3   "   "
                        16-20   "   "   £4   "   "

All available from
LUPUS UK, St James House, Eastern Road, Romford, Essex, RM1 3NH

Notes

Notes

Notes